INJURY TIME

INJURY TIME

A NOVEL BY

Beryl Bainbridge

GEORGE BRAZILLER

NEW YORK

Published in the United States in 1977
by George Braziller, Inc.
Copyright © 1977 by Beryl Bainbridge
Originally published in Great Britain
by Gerald Duckworth & Co. Ltd.

Library of Congress Cataloging in Publication Data

Bainbridge, Beryl, 1933–
  Injury time.

  I. Title.
PZ4.B162In   1977   [PR6052.A3195]   823'.9'14   77–21127
ISBN: 0–8076–0881–5

Printed in the United States of America
FIRST AMERICAN EDITION

FOR PSICHE AND PHILIP HUGHES WITH LOVE

1

During the partners' lunch, old Gifford talked
indistinctly about the Rawlinson account: something to do with the new man on the board not
having a first-class brain—he didn't come up to
scratch. From time to time Gifford's shoulder
dipped below the level of the tablecloth; he
seemed to have dropped something. Hatters,
from the Overseas department, told a story in-
volving a doctor and a woman patient who heard
pop music whenever her husband made love to
her. Edward Freeman, who was seated opposite,
missed the punch line. The fellow appeared to be
muttering, or perhaps his own hearing was at
fault. Alarmed by this new defect—lately he had
been forced to wear spectacles when attempting

the crossword—he stuck his finger in his ear and waggled it vigorously back and forth. Hatters, flourishing his fork in the air, was saying quite clearly that the engine of his car needed tuning. Edward allowed Mrs. Chalmers to serve him with a second helping of lamb; he wasn't hungry but he contributed twenty pounds a month toward the cost of the office lunches and was damned if he was letting a penny of it go to waste. Binny said it was killing him, all that meat stewed in wine and all those puddings consumed every day of the week. "Men of your age," she constantly warned him, "are at risk. You'll have a heart attack." At this moment, with less than six hours to go before the dinner party, he felt that a small coronary might do him the world of good. He didn't think Binny would visit him in hospital— she wasn't malicious. He could just lie there for several days, undergoing tests, doing a spot of reading, trying to sort himself out.

Even so, when lunch was over he took the lift to his office and denied himself the exertion of climbing three flights of stairs. The telephone rang as he came through the door. It was his wife Helen.

"Are you going to be very late tonight?" she asked. "Or just late?"

"Oh, I shan't be late," he said. "I mean, I'll try to get away early."

"You usually try," she said.

There was a slight pause. Edward looked at the

photograph of her, framed in leather, on the windowsill. She was holding a baby. On his desk was a snapshot of the same baby, several years older, crouched in a blurred garden cradling a rabbit in his arms.

"You see," she said, "if I leave my meeting early and you don't get back for hours, it's a bit of a waste of effort . . . on my part. Do you see what I mean?"

"Yes," he said. "But I shouldn't think old Simpson will want to hang on too long. Not with his leg."

"That's true enough."

"Look here," he said desperately. "Better be on the safe side. One can never tell with old Simpson. I suppose I could be late . . . I don't want to spoil your meeting. I don't want you to scamper away only to find I've got caught up."

"All right then, dear," she said. "I won't."

When she'd rung off he felt aggrieved. He wasn't always late, not every night. Tuesday for instance he never visited Binny, and hardly ever on a Thursday. That was the night her youngest daughter went to Brownies and was inclined to be boisterous afterwards. And what about those numerous occasions when he'd made a special effort to get home early, left his evening post unsigned, faced the frightful rush-hour traffic and arrived in time to catch Helen backing down the path in the Mini, gadding off to yet another meeting? She wasn't the only one who could imply there was cause for complaint, not by any means.

The telephone rang again. He knew at once it was Binny, because when he said Hello there was no reply, merely a sort of offended breathing. There had evidently been some deficiency of feeling in his voice when he first greeted her, a degree of casualness that she hadn't liked. "Hello, Hello," he persisted. He kept his eyes fixed on the snapshot of the rabbit struggling in his son's arms. He couldn't remember what they'd called the animal . . . Tiger? . . . Twinkle? The beastly thing had turned the garden into a waste land before dying of old age and being shovelled under the damson tree.

"Look here," he lied. "I'm frightfully busy. May I ring you back?"

"Don't bother," said Binny, and put down the receiver.

He dialled her number immediately. She made him wait at least half a minute before answering. "Look, don't be angry," he pleaded. "I had somebody in my room."

"Oh yes."

"You don't seem to realize I'm a very busy man. I had poor old Woodford with me."

"What's poor about him?"

"They're leaving him with nothing," Edward said. "The Inland Revenue are bleeding him white."

"What do you call nothing?" demanded Binny.

He knew he shouldn't get involved in this sort

of discussion—he always came off the worse for wear and was apt to be indiscreet about clients' accounts. "They're taking eighty-three pence in the pound," he confided, voice thin with outrage.

"If they take that much," said Binny, "he must be rolling. It still leaves him with seventeen p and if he's paying supertax I bet the seventeen p's jolly well add up. You can hardly expect me to pass round the hat."

They dwelt on old Woodford's tax problems, loudly, for quite some time. Edward found her tone of voice offensive. After all, he'd taken a considerable risk in agreeing to invite Simpson and his wife to dinner at Binny's house. He hadn't so much agreed as been goaded into the arrangement. Binny had intimated in her forthright way that she was sick to death of being introduced only to those boozy male acquaintances of his who thought he was a hell of a dog for getting his leg over. She wanted to meet his real friends, preferably a married couple. "I'm not going to be hidden in the shadows of the saloon bar any longer," she'd said. She was perfectly within her rights, of course. It was rotten for her, reeling out of the dentist alone, unable to depend upon him at Christmas, forced to see him at times mostly convenient to Helen. He gave her so little; he denied her the simple pleasures a wife took for granted—that business of cooking his meals, remembering his sister's birthday, putting intricate little bundles of socks into his drawer. All he had to offer were those pitifully few hours of an evening, if and when Helen chose to go to one of her meetings.

And life, as Binny so often observed, was perilously short. She'd remarked upon it the first time they met, at a wine and cheese party given by clients of his—a firm of estate agents in Chalk Farm. He was early and knew no one save the senior partner, and was smarting because Helen had refused to accompany him; she preferred instead to attend an Inter Action group in Hampstead where she sometimes knelt on the floor and stroked people seated on either side. It was his impression afterwards that, when he entered the estate agents' office, he'd noticed a pale and diminutive woman standing by the window. She wore a bunch of artificial flowers pinned to the collar of her dress and it was these same limp violets that enabled him later, much later, when she'd maneuvered him behind a filing cabinet, to identify Binny. During the evening she had unaccountably gained weight and color from somewhere. Her eyes shone brilliantly. She kept asking him if he was happy. It was then, just as he began to feel undeniably cheerful—he heard his own laughter loud above the murmur of voices—that she spoke of death, likening middle age to the second half of a football match. The game, she said, long since decided, was drawing to a close. Short of breath and flecked with mud, trembling in every limb, the players struggled up and down the pitch,

8

waiting for the final whistle to blow. "Although I am still active in mid field," she told him, "it may be that I won't play to the end. It's possible that I shall be sent off." "Ah no," he cried, filled with a tenderness that was surely out of place after so short an acquaintanceship. "Not you." But Binny hadn't heard him. She said she herself had enjoyed a life packed full of incident. She wondered if others could say the same. He was aware that as she talked the tips of her fingers brushed his own. She had travelled extensively in Europe, been divorced, known many lovers. Suddenly depressed, he longed to go home and watch television. He tried to catch the attention of the senior partner, and failed. Binny swayed a little on her feet and leaned against him; the violets rustled on her breast. He escorted her to a terraced house in Fulton Street and fell over a bicycle in the hall. Shaken by her acceptance of death, he confessed that the passage of time affected him in a retrospective sort of way. He didn't fear the deterioration that old age might bring—increased blood pressure, varicose veins, palpitations of the heart. It was waking in the night, as he did frequently, from dreams clear in every detail, of gardens glimpsed from windows, roads travelled, rooms dwelt in as a boy, that caused him agitation. He regretted that he no longer experienced the present or looked forward to the future. Unusually articulate and rubbing his shin bone, bruised from contact with the mudguard in the hall, he would have confided more but felt he was becoming boring. She made him a cup of coffee and enlisted his help with her tax problems, crying out in the middle of his discourse upon capital growth and percentages that she needed to embrace him. Remembering her formidable list of lovers, he was concerned she might be riddled with disease. He evaded her outstretched arms and circled the living room. As he walked, his life flew with him—the edge of a sports-field one day in summer, his father's hand scuttling into a leather glove, the glimmer of a prefect's badge lying in an oblong of sunlight on a desk—at last, desperate to blot out the shrill blast of that final whistle, he knelt at Binny's feet and crawled with her on to the dusty sofa.

He thought possibly it was the unsatisfactory briefness of his moments with Binny that explained his continuing desire to see her. God knows, she was rude enough to him, but then they spent so little time together that her insulting behavior never had a chance to build up into anything sufficiently awful; she never actually hit him. She was too often interrupted by the children, who were either in and using the telephone, or out and telephoning in. They were always being flung out of poolrooms or cafés, or held at railway stations for the non-payment of fares. Once the youngest child's hampster started to die the moment Edward entered the house. Edward had been required to spoon brandy down the animal's throat until it passed on. The sight of those delicate paws, tipped with pink, feebly scratching the air, reminded Edward of his own inner conflict. There were some doors that would never open. Binny was a wonderful mother, but she didn't seem to realize he was a very busy man and his time was limited. They could never do anything until her ten-year-old had settled down for the night. They could usually start doing something at about five to eleven, and then they had to do it very quickly because Edward had to leave at quarter past eleven. He was always whispering frantically into Binny's ear what he might do if only they had a whole evening together, and she grew quite pale and breathless and hugged him fearfully tightly in the hall, mostly when seeing him out. He loved her when she had difficulty in breathing. Just thinking about it made him feel disturbed.

Binny was telling him in a hectoring manner that she bet old Woodford, despite extreme poverty, had two cars and a mansion in the country.

He said bitterly, "I wish to God the Simpsons weren't coming to dinner tonight. I wish we were on our own." In order to ensure a peaceful evening without undue excitement, for the first time in all the years he had known her the children were spending the night elsewhere.

"I'm not calling it dinner," said Binny ominously.

"Oh, aren't you?" he said.

"No, I'm bloody well not."

"Well, what are you calling it?" he asked uneasily.

Evidently she was worried about the food she was preparing. She had telephoned, most likely, to ask him if the menu she had decided upon was suitable, and that first insensitively expressed Hello of his had depressed her. He didn't think she was a very good cook—not that she'd ever made him a meal—but he sensed that her attitude to food was rather casual. When he took her out to dinner quite normal things, like artichokes, annoyed her. She said they were a waste of time. He hadn't actually spotted two plates in her kitchen with the same pattern round the rim. However, none of that counted at the moment. She could burn every morsel to be eaten and dispense entirely with knives and forks, if only the evening passed without repercussions. It was vital that nobody dropped in. He longed to ask Binny if she had taken precautions against such an event, but he knew her reply would be deliberately calculated to alarm. She would probably inform him she was hauling up the drawbridge any moment now, but could he tell her anything about the little man on the corner in the mackintosh, the one with the binoculars and the camera. He hadn't met Simpson's wife before, but he was fairly certain there was no danger there. He gathered that Simpson's wife had once studied Esperanto, and Simpson boasted that she regularly visited the local pub with a girl friend. She was obviously pretty broadminded and not the sort to go round telling everyone he was carrying on with another woman. But what if a neighbor of Binny's dropped in during the meal and turned out to be a friend of a mutual friend? Possibly a friend of the girl who went to the pub with Simpson's wife. And what if they happened to know someone who went to the same Liberal party meetings as Helen or employed the same cleaning lady? It could get back. People were always remarking on the smallness of the world since the invention of the airplane.

Dreadfully agitated, Edward shuffled the papers on his desk and thought he experienced a sharp pain in his chest.

"What's up with you?" asked Binny. "What did you make that noise for?"

He denied that he had made any noise out of the ordinary. There was silence for several seconds until Binny said he was to stop worrying about being caught out. He protested it was the last thing on his mind.

"Liar," she cried exultantly. "You're scared rigid someone will tell your wife. You didn't have to come to dinner, you know."

"But I want to come to dinner—"

"Nobody forced you. Nobody pulled your toenails out."

He insisted he was looking forward to the evening ahead and Binny said like hell he was and she didn't understand the way his mind worked; he was completely foreign to her, complaining on the one hand that until they met he had found his life dull, sordid—

"Not sordid," he objected. "My life has never been sordid."

"Well, squalid, then. You were bothered about growing old."

"Whereas now," he observed sharply, "I doubt if I'll live that long."

It seemed to put her in a better mood, his fear of untimely death. She laughed a lot and told him he was lovely and that if he was very good she wouldn't argue with him for a whole week.

When he put the phone down his hands were trembling.

2

Binny was disturbed in the middle of washing down the paintwork in the kitchen by the arrival of her friend Alma Waterhouse who had come in a taxi to borrow the hoover.

It was an awkward situation with the meter ticking over.

"It won't work," improvised Binny. "Someone's taken the plug off the end."

Alma went into the street to send the taxi man away. Binny dragged the hoover from under the stairs and threw it down the back steps into the yard. It wouldn't do to let Alma know that she herself wanted to use the machine. It would arouse suspicion. Binny rarely hoovered. If she admitted that guests were coming for the evening, Alma would expect to be invited. She was having husband trouble and needed taking out of herself.

On the draining-board glittered four cooking apples, stuffed with raisins and wrapped in silver foil. Hastily bundling them into a shopping bag, Binny dropped them behind the fridge. Alma returned. She took from the pocket of her camel coat a quarter bottle of whisky and approached the cupboard where the glasses were kept.

"I can't allow it," said Binny. Defiantly she barred the way.

"Whatever's the matter?" cried Alma, astonished at her attitude. "We could do with a little swiggie, darling. It's awfully cold out." Alma was a great believer in swiggies, whatever the temperature.

Binny stood her ground and adopted a crucified position against the mahogany wall cupboard. She gazed seriously at Alma and after a pause added the words "Not now," holding aloft a pink sponge with which she had rinsed the woodwork; lukewarm water trickled down her arm. Impressed, Alma stepped back and put away the bottle. Binny said she had shopping to do. She tied a scarf over her newly washed hair and pushed Alma out of the house, striding ahead along the alleyway toward the High Street. Behind the wire netting of the play center, children crawled along concrete pipes, screaming.

"Have I said anything out of turn?" asked

Alma, teetering over the cobblestones in her high-heeled boots.

Binny was feeling terribly emotional. She wished she hadn't spoken so harshly to Edward on the telephone and regretted she'd been unkind about his friend, old Woodford. It wasn't very nice, the government taking his money off him like that. She wouldn't like it. It was the way Edward *hadn't* said Hello that had put a damper on things. She'd been in perfectly good spirits when dialling his number. She'd scrubbed the bath, hung clean towels over the edge and done all that raisin business with the apples. Then quite suddenly, on hearing his clipped and well-bred voice, she had dropped into somewhere dark and confined—she was shut inside a box beneath a river. She felt he wouldn't be able to hear her even if she shouted. This feeling of being locked away from him had something to do with visualizing Edward, on the other end of the telephone, leaning against a desk polished by somebody he had never met, blotting the corners of his mouth to remove traces of a meal he hadn't cooked, with a handkerchief that came fresh and laundered out of his breast pocket as if by magic. It was the privileged style in which the man lived that silenced her.

When she'd first seen him, stepping through the doorway of the outer office in Chalk Farm, he'd reminded her of various portly relatives glimpsed only in the pages of photograph albums.

He wore galoshes and held, either in his hand or teeth, the stem of a small and blackened pipe. His face, which was pale and fair, had a curious swelling between the eyebrows as though he had been stung by an insect. Bitten by life, she thought, watching his mouth open and close behind a drift of tobacco smoke. The way he told it, there wasn't much point to his existence. He had always done the right thing, supported his wife, educated his son, made sure the garden was tidy. There had been that trouble years ago—here he waved his hand rather vaguely in the air as if turning the handle of a gramophone—but he had learned to live with it. Binny pretended at first she was still married, to avoid complications. But later in the evening, rather charmed by those galoshes and the manner in which he constantly puffed, sucked and fooled over his pipe, she allowed him to see her home. He kept looking at himself in the mirror. She couldn't be sure if the swelling upon his forehead made him appear hideous, or distinguished in a Roman sort of way. She couldn't tell at all now because, loving him as she supposed she did, she no longer saw him as he was. That first night he had spoken confusedly of his time at boarding school. Captain of the cricket team . . . head of his dormitory . . . That rotter Jonas . . . If it hadn't been for Muldoon—what a stinker *he'd* turned out to be. He was obviously re-living the heyday of his prep school years. There was something too about his father and a pair of gloves, and a beastly rumpus over a prefect's badge. She could make little sense of it. Having attended grammar school and forgotten all about it, Binny was touched by his continued preoccupation with those far-off boyhood days.

If she hadn't been touched, she thought gloomily, she wouldn't be out in this weather, catering for his friends.

On the pavement outside the British Rail warehouse, lying in disorder across the rusted springs of a double bed, sprawled several elderly men and women drinking out of a communal bottle. Binny retraced her steps and caught hold of Alma's arm.

"It's everywhere," she whispered. "Where are the police?"

"Don't talk nonsense," scolded Alma. "The last thing we need is a policeman."

Smiling and nodding ingratiatingly, she led Binny forward. An old woman in a fur coat and a pair of tennis shoes, reclining on one elbow as though in a punt on a lake, stared at Alma in admiration. "My goodness," she shouted. "You're a bonny girl. Will you look at that hair on her head?" Alma's hair, rinsed to an unusual shade of strawberry blonde, was blowing in all directions.

Pleased, Alma stopped and confessed it wasn't altogether natural. "I use a little something," she confided. "Hint of a Tint . . . every second or third wash."

Bouncing in excitement on the dilapidated bed, unsettling her geriatric companions wrapped in sacking, the old woman laughed and leered her approval. Two men struggled upright into a sitting position and spat violently into the gutter. Their eyes, half averted, were those of animals existing in darkness. Binny ran away, and emerged breathlessly on to the High Street looking for someone in authority.

"You're a bundle of nerves," decided Alma some moments later, coming across Binny leaning against the wall of a public house. "You should have had a little swiggie when I pressed you."

"I don't know how you could talk to them," said Binny. "They looked dangerous."

"Silly girl. They were only enjoying themselves."

"She had iodine dabbed all over her face," said Binny.

"Well, she had one or two cuts on her nose," defended Alma. "It's natural. Old people are always falling over. Think of your own mother when she dislocated her hip."

"She stumbled getting out of a taxi," Binny said. "She wasn't rolling about in the gutter with a bottle of booze."

In silence they walked down the street. Alma slowed her steps expectantly at each shop doorway, but Binny hurried on. She had no money.

At last, made miserable by the chill wind and deafened by the roar of traffic, they fled inside the Wimpy bar for a cup of coffee. The waitress was affronted at the bold way they expected service. After five minutes of hostile inactivity she relented and left two cups of pale yellow liquid at the edge of the table.

"I wouldn't mind a doughnut," called Alma, but the waitress had better things to do.

From where she sat in the window, Binny could see both the perambulator braked at the steps of the bank and the clock above the door of the shoe shop. It was ten minutes to three. If the bank closed before she had time to cash her check, she wouldn't be able to afford cream for the baked apples, or Greek bread, or buy enough salad to make a splash. She was tempting fate. She wanted the dinner party to go well for Edward's sake, but she didn't want to strive for success. All her life she had found that when she went to a great deal of trouble, the results were never satisfactory; her greatest triumphs had been accidental.

A man in a bowler hat, strolling backwards and forwards in front of the bank, took a rolled-up newspaper from under his arm, and pausing in his stride proceeded to tap the hood of the perambulator.

Alma was in the middle of a story concerning her son Victor, who only the day before had behaved badly in a car. "He told me to throw it away," she was explaining. "He said the smoke irritated his throat. So I did. Not at once, I grant you—after a few quick puffs. I know it's not fair to give the young cancer. We'd been for an Indian meal. I opened the window and threw it out and he told me to shut the window. He jostled me. Then he called me a toe-rag."

A thin woman in a mackintosh came out of the doorway of the National Westminster and stood for a moment looking at the traffic. The bowler-hatted man dropped his newspaper onto the hood of the pram and walked briskly away.

"Look at that," said Binny, pointing. She watched him disappear into the entrance of the tube station.

"Don't be fickle, darling," reproved Alma. "You be content with your lovely Teddy." She was keen on Edward and he liked her, though he was not overfond of being called Ted.

The woman in the mackintosh descended the steps of the bank awkwardly, as though afraid she might lose her balance. Using her stomach to propel the pram, she picked up the rolled newspaper and tipped it over the edge of the storm shield.

"Poor little thing," cried Binny, aloud. It was unthinkable that any mother should shove a dirty newspaper on to the pillow of a sleeping child. The world was menacing and full of alarms. "I can't stand it," she told Alma. "It's disgusting and frightening."

"What is?" asked Alma, gazing in bewilderment at the plastic table top and the sauce bottle in the shape of a tomato, a crust like blood rimming the imitation stalk.

"Anywhere you can possibly go," said Binny.

"It's waiting round the corner. Faces with scabs . . . hit-and-run drivers . . ."

Though most of her life she had rushed headlong into danger and excitement, she had travelled first-class, so to speak, with a carriage attendant within call. The world was less predictable now. The guard was on strike and the communication cord had been ripped from the roof. It wasn't the same. In her day dreams, usually accompanied by a panic-stricken Edward, she was always being blown up in airplanes or going down in ships.

"There, there," soothed Alma, taking Binny's hand and patting it. "It's probably the change that's upsetting you, darling." And indeed Binny's normally pale cheeks flamed a deep and fierce red.

"I can't help noticing details," said Binny. "Little clues and suchlike. I'd like to switch over, but I can't."

Alma looked at her.

"I keep thinking I'm watching television," Binny said. "There doesn't seem to be much difference." She stared mesmerized out of the window.

Alma asked for the bill and said she'd phone in the morning to see if Binny felt more settled. Better still, she could call round this evening for a little chat.

"No," said Binny. "I shall go to bed early." At this lie her face flushed more than ever. "But I doubt if it will do any good. I don't know how you can be so blind. The whole world's changed. It's not my little change that's making the difference." Seeing that Alma appeared unconvinced she added, "I don't suppose you called *your* mother a toe-rag."

Alma agreed she hadn't, but then in their day the world had been unknown. "Old cow," she admitted. "Or flipping swine. I got my face slapped." She touched her cheek at the memory.

"I said bugger once," recalled Binny. "I said it to a chair in Mother's bedroom and she overheard. She said a policeman would come round and wash my mouth out."

"You're always looking for policemen," said Alma thoughtfully. She looked at the bill and was astonished at the service charge.

"I wonder," asked Binny, "if we should hit the children more?" She never had, not even when they punched her or broke something valuable. When she was younger she would have argued to the death that it was wrong to beat a child. Now she wasn't so sure. Somewhere along the line mistakes had been made: the way everyone accepted those telephone calls in the night from the police holding the children in the cells for disorderly behavior; the way the children lolled about the house, refusing to go out until the pubs opened. She had started with such liberal leftish ideas upon most things—education, socialism, capital punishment, sex and so forth—and then, like an old and tired horse knowing the road home, had veered inexorably to the right. Only the other day her son had called her a fascist pig. It was true she didn't want to share anything any more, particularly not with the children.

"You are in a state," Alma said. "Perhaps you need a little holiday."

"You know I can't leave the children," said Binny hastily. Alma was always trying to get her to go on little holidays. Binny had accompanied her once to Brighton for three days and returned practically an alcoholic. Last summer Alma had wanted her to fly on a package deal to Tunisia. She said it was very cheap and would do her the world of good. Binny hadn't gone. Alma had come home with a stubborn case of crabs which she said she'd caught off a camel.

"I must get on," said Binny, worriedly, rising from her seat, thinking at this rate she wouldn't reach the bank before nightfall.

They kissed and parted outside Boots the chemist. Alma decided to wait for a taxi. Trying to keep warm, she hopped cheerfully from one leg to another, shouting Goodbye repeatedly above the din of traffic, as though for the very last time.

Binny went into the bank. In the queue at the cashier's counter waited a thin woman in a mackintosh. Binny was so surprised she darted back to the door and looked outside. Perhaps the baby was parked in a side street—after all those warnings about leaving children unattended! She walked down the steps, though it was none of her business, and round the corner. There was no sign of a pram. The wind tore at her clothes. She thought she saw familiar faces, framed in windows, flickering past her as the cars swarmed toward the High Street. Confused, she raised her arm in greeting, imagining she heard above the fluttering of her headscarf a voice crying her name. "I'm all at sea," she said out loud and, trying not to tremble, returned to the bank.

The woman was now third in line at the cashier's grill. Binny couldn't see her face. She had short colorless hair, and gray stockings with a seam, and she carried a plastic shopping bag. At the counter, the fishmonger from Barretts, two fingers clumsy with sticking plaster, was stacking cellophane packets of small change into a hold-all. As he struggled with the zip of the canvas bag, the woman slipped from her place in the queue and joined the end of a third line of customers further along the counter. She looked directly at Binny. Forty years earlier, behind a wall and across the road from Binny's house, there had stood a home for fallen girls. On Sundays, with heads grotesquely shaven to eliminate lice, the inmates formed in twos upon the pavement. In the bold eyes of the woman, Binny recalled instantly the glances of those other, indecent girls, bobbing beneath the branches of almond trees in bloom, swaying, with fragile necks exposed like stalks of flowers in a brutal crocodile to church. She blushed.

When she had cashed her check and was out in the street, she found that the noise and the cold no longer bothered her. Something had pleased her, raised her spirits, though what it was she couldn't be sure. She bought the bread she needed and a carton of double cream. She swept in and out of shops and didn't complain when various men jumped the queue and were served out of turn. She was able to smile quite charitably, after she had leapt to safety, at a youth on a bicycle who failed to run her down on the zebra crossing.

3

Edward met old Simpson for a drink in the Hare and Hounds. The place was filled with tired businessmen pepping themselves up before returning home.

"I see no reason why you shouldn't claim a certain proportion for entertainment," said Edward. "None at all. Providing you can produce the restaurant bills."

"Quite so," agreed Simpson.

"But I don't feel we can justifiably put forward your wife's hairdressing expenses. Not for the golf club night and so forth. It's not strictly business. See what I mean?"

"Yes," said Simpson, disappointed.

"I mean, it's not as if she's a hostess in a night

club, for instance. Or a television personality."

"I may have misled you about the wife," Simpson said. "She's not altogether sympatico to this evening."

"Good Lord," cried Edward, instantly alarmed. "I thought you said she was a woman of the world?"

"She's that of course," said Simpson. "But the way she sees it, it's a bit not on."

"She will come, won't she?" asked Edward. He felt like hitting old Simpson between the eyes with his fist. All that rubbish he'd talked about it being a bit of a lark and what a terrific sport the old woman was.

"The way she sees it," explained Simpson, "it's definitely a bit tricky. How would you like it if Helen was meeting some fellow on the side and she asked me round to your house to meet him?"

It seemed to Edward a highly unlikely situation, knowing what Helen thought about Simpson and fellows in general, but he nodded his head and pretended Simpson had a point there.

"Put it another way," Simpson went on. "What if my wife asked you and your lady friend to dinner behind my back? I trust you'd refuse."

"Need you ask?" Edward said.

"I don't want you to run away with the idea that the wife's narrow. She's not, believe you me. I'll tell you a little story. Keep it under your hat; I shouldn't like it to go any further. She got a proposition from a mutual friend of ours—well, wife of a friend of mine, as a matter of fact. Let's call her X. X phoned the wife and said could she come round and talk to her—"

"Whose wife?" asked Edward.

"Mine, of course," said Simpson. "It was absolutely vital that Y shouldn't get to know—"

"I don't quite follow you," said Edward, mystified by Simpson's alphabetical acquaintances. "Did your wife tell you she'd been propositioned?"

"Don't be dense," cried Simpson testily. "My wife wasn't propositioned. X was."

"Yes, of course." Edward nodded. He didn't want to antagonize Simpson, not when Binny's dinner party hung in the balance. At this moment, he no longer cared about himself and the possibility of being caught out. He thought only of Binny, slaving over a hot stove. "Stupid of me," he admitted. "It's my training, I suppose. Making sure the figures add up . . . that sort of thing. Do go on."

"It seems," continued Simpson, "that X was carrying on with Z. Had been for quite some time. Met him at a masonic do last year. Upshot of it was, X wanted the wife to lend out our spare room for the afternoon."

"Good God," murmured Edward. Though he had lost track of X and Z and was totally foxed by Y, he did sympathize with their general predicament.

"The wife handled it rather cleverly, I

thought," said Simpson. "She said they could have the room but would they please wash the sheets out afterwards, or leave money on the table for laundering. And would they keep the window and the door open."

"The window?" said Edward. He thought Simpson's wife must have a peculiarly coarse sense of humor. Or possibly she was a voyeur.

"Took all the romance out of it," cried Simpson with satisfaction. "Exposed it for what it was. Put the kibosh on it, no two ways about it."

"Goodness, yes," said Edward, though it seemed to him, once they had come to some agreement about being spied upon, a small enough price to pay for a whole afternoon of love.

He fought his way to the counter and ordered another two pints of beer and waited, pipe clamped in his mouth like a dummy, craning upwards to see his reflection in the mirror above the bar. He needed a haircut; a pale forelock dangled over one eye. He would have gone to the barber's days ago—he'd noticed a few raised eyebrows in the office—but Binny had once remarked she liked men with untidy heads. He thought his forelock made him look rather boyish. Binny referred to it sometimes as a fetlock. At others, when she'd taken a glass or two of wine, she called it his foreskin. He'd better watch Binny's intake tonight—he didn't feel Simpson's wife would go for that kind of table talk. Always supposing she intended to be present. What on earth was he going to tell Binny if the Simpsons backed out at this late hour? She'd sounded so argumentative on the telephone, though at the end she'd said he was lovely. She did care for him. She gave him her love mostly without trying to bind him, without endangering his marriage. It was true there'd been a few unfortunate lapses, like the weekend she'd rung his house from some drinking club in Soho. He'd answered the phone himself, thank God, but it was frightfully tricky, standing in the hall in his pajamas in the middle of the night trying to convey through references to tax returns that he loved her, fearful of Helen on the landing listening to every word. There had been too that incident when he couldn't see Binny because he wanted to prune his roses, and she'd threatened to come round in the night and set fire to his garden. Later, a small corner of the lawn had been found mysteriously singed, but nothing had ever been proved. In the beginning he had fallen in love with her because she advised him they must live each day as if it was their last: bearing in mind that any moment the final whistle could blow, it was pointless to spoil the time they had left with the making of impossible demands. "You don't want to leave your wife," she'd said. "And I don't want you to." But as the months passed and she made various disparaging remarks about married men and their duplicity, it occurred to him that possibly this was precisely what she required of him. It made him very uncomfortable. He tried once to bring the subject into the open. "We could be jolly happy," he supposed. "We'd drink far too much and go to bed in the afternoon"—Helen disapproved of the afternoon—"if we lived together." Glaring at him as though he'd uttered a racist remark and snapping her rather large white teeth, Binny had cried, "You must be mad. Stark raving mad."

It was confusing for him. He obviously served some purpose in her life. Often he was reminded of a Punch and Judy show he had watched on the sands at Eastbourne when he was a child. Hearing that nasal voice screaming above the incoming tide, "Who's a naughty boy, then?," and flinching at the sound of those repeated blows to the head, he had not understood what was expected of him. Clutching his bucket and spade, he hadn't known whether to laugh or cry.

Binny could be so cold when standing up and facing him, or shouting at him down the telephone, and so warm when lying in his arms. When he thought of those snatched perspiring moments on the sofa, the bathroom floor, the divan bed in Binny's back room, he felt he could forgive her anything and dreamed of devoting the rest of his life to making her happy.

He paid for the drinks and returned to the table. He looked down at Simpson's balding crown and said firmly, "Look here, old man. What's the form tonight? You are coming, I take it?"

"Good Lord, yes," said Simpson. "I wouldn't miss it for worlds."

"What about the wife?"

"We're both coming," Simpson said. "Depend on it. I just wanted to warn you it might be a bit sticky at first. Muriel might be a shade off-hand. But she'll thaw." He patted Edward's knee encouragingly.

"You may find it a little bohemian tonight," said Edward. "Just a bit."

"Christ," cried Simpson. "I feared as much. Muriel won't stand for it, you know."

"I meant domestically," Edward said. "Space-wise, facilities . . . knives and forks. See what I mean?"

"Oh," said Simpson. "Rough and ready, is that it?"

"A little," Edward said, feeling disloyal. "Binny's not one for appearances."

"Say no more." Simpson nodded sympathetically. "Are you going home to change?"

"No," said Edward. "It's a shade awkward getting out again. I thought I might go back to the office and sign a little post."

Simpson suggested Edward should come home with him for a wash-and-brush-up. Then they could all arrive together.

Edward accepted. "Have you mentioned to your wife," he said, "that we're supposed to have met? Her and me. Binny particularly stressed that

I should invite close mutual friends."

"Don't push it, old boy," advised Simpson with some irritation. 'It's been difficult enough to persuade her to sit down with you, let alone pretend you've been friendly for years. And you'd better watch the hanky panky."

"Hanky panky?"

"Touching . . . fooling about . . . any outward show. Muriel won't like it."

"I have to be home by eleven," said Edward. "I don't think there'll be time for hanky panky."

No further mention was made of his going back with Simpson for a wash. After a quarter of an hour Simpson got up to go and said he'd see him in the trenches at twenty hundred hours. He nudged Edward in the ribs. "Synchronize watches . . . we'll go over the top together." Laughing heartily and thinking what a bloody ass the man was, Edward said goodbye. He bought a packet of cashew nuts to tide himself over until dinner, and on an unfortunate impulse telephoned Binny.

"What do you want?" she asked.

"Nothing really. I've just been chatting to old Simpson. He was a bit foolish, I thought."

"How surprising!"

"I meant he spoke rather childishly. He's not as broadminded as one thinks."

"What's all that noise?" Binny said. "Where are you?"

"In the office," he lied. "Simpson said what would I think if Helen asked him and his wife round for a meal."

"What are you on about? I thought they'd had dozens of meals at your house?"

"I'm not explaining myself very clearly," he said. "I get the feeling he doesn't approve of . . . well, you know . . ."

"I don't know," she snapped. "Spit it out."

"Us," he said lamely. "Carrying on."

She fell silent. Edward ground the receiver so tightly against his ear, to drown the pub sounds all around him, that his eyes began to water.

"You told me he'd been to a V.D. clinic," said Binny finally.

Oh God, he thought, had he really confided that? She'd probably bring it up at dinner if things went badly. "Well, yes," he said. "But there was never anything actually wrong."

"Who the hell does he think he is? He's in no position to object to anybody carrying on."

"I think," said Edward, "that it's his wife more than him."

"I'll bet it is," Binny crowed. "She probably feels that if you're doing it, then her old Simpson's at it too."

"You are clever," he said tenderly. "I do love you, you know."

"Like bloody hell," she said, and told him she must get on.

She was a mystery to him; she had no small talk at all.

He returned to the office. Here he began to compose a fairly resentful letter to Simpson, indicating that he thought it inadvisable to claim such and such an amount for the cleaning of his business premises ". . . It would seem to me, in the circumstances, an unrealistic and preposterous sum, more in keeping with maintaining the hygienic standards of a research laboratory than a spare parts factory, and one which the Inspector of Taxes would undoubtedly and deservedly view with suspicion, etc., etc. . . ."

4

Binny laid the dining-room table, still wearing
her headscarf and outdoor coat. Underneath she
had changed into her best black dress. The table
was situated in the front half of the ground-floor
room. The back half contained the kitchen. In it
was a stove, a fridge and a very small draining-
board. So great was Binny's abhorrence of cooking that she'd torn down the shelving and plastic
work surfaces installed by a previous owner and
stacked everything—food, crockery, pans—into
an article of furniture she called a wall cupboard.
It was, in reality, a gentleman's wardrobe, still
fragrant with the smell of Havana cigars, complete with little compartments for starched and
detachable collars in which Binny kept the knives

and forks. From the back window there was a view of a yard, a brick wall, and a rabbit hutch that Edward had given her.

Moving about the table, cheerful and organized, Binny was interrupted by her daughter, Lucy, who was eighteen and dressed as though ready for work on a building site.

"Screw me," cried Lucy, smiling for once, eyeing the cut flowers and the folded napkins. "Having a knees-up, are we?" She had known for days that Binny was expecting guests, but she liked to tease. She seized her mother by the shoulders and shook her. Binny's headscarf slithered over her eyes. "Who's a posh girl, then?"

"Don't, darling," said Binny.

Lucy flung herself sideways on to the sofa, crushing the newly plumped cushions. She began to roll a cigarette. She said critically, "I should wear something more suitable, if I were you. They'll think you're not stopping."

Binny noticed that her daughter's army boots, heavily studded, were scuffing a carpet already flecked with pieces of cotton thread and bits of fluff. It had started to rain when she'd returned from the bank and she hadn't felt like going down into the yard to retrieve the hoover. The inside might have got wet and she didn't want to risk being electrocuted. Perhaps no one would notice the carpet once the drink started going down.

"I think, darling," said Binny, "you'd better be off. If that's all right with you. Just pop the baby into the Evans', there's a good girl."

The baby, who was almost eleven years old, was quite capable of climbing the fence and going up the steps to the house next door, but Binny worried.

"Where's big-dick?" asked Lucy.

"Behave," pleaded Binny. She counted inwardly to ten and busied herself with titivating the table. Her son Gregory, bribed with a pound note, was, she hoped, half-way across London on the underground, bound for the house of his friend Adam.

Lucy appeared to have fallen asleep. Cigarette papers and grains of tobacco littered her chest. "Will you get up?" said Binny. "At once. Please, dear."

There was very little left for her to do. She'd peeled the potatoes, washed the lettuce, sprinkled herb things on the meat. Still, she wanted her daughters out of the way. Being constantly with the children was like wearing a pair of shoes that were expensive and too small. She couldn't bear to throw them out, but they gave her blisters. It would be nice having Edward in the house with other people present. Adults. She could talk about things without having to explain herself, without endlessly repeating what she'd said in the first place. No one would interrupt her with requests for jam, or money for the bus. Nobody would tell her to shut up. She liked Edward when he'd had a lot to drink. His eyes, bloodshot and sleepy, gazed at her with passion. She would be able to lean against him and give him the biggest lamb chop. When he went into the bathroom he would notice how clean the bowl was and the basin. She knew it was important to him that the house should look like a good investment.

"Lucy," she said loudly. "It's almost seven o'clock."

"Rubbish," Lucy said. "It can't be. We'd have heard Mrs. Papastavrou." Across the street was a post-war block of flats, lit at night like a ship on its maiden voyage and totally deserted by day. The rent collector and the man from the Providential were seen to walk along the concrete balconies, but the inmates remained hidden. The exception was Mrs. Papastavrou, an elderly Greek now living on the top floor, who had originally occupied a flat on the ground floor and been carried aloft, out of harm's way, after knifing the lady who brought the meals-on-wheels. Mrs. Papastavrou had grown frail and thin before the wounding. Her tray was collected with the food untouched on her plate. In an effort to stimulate her appetite the Council provided her with stuffed vine leaves and cartons of taramasalata. Thinking she was being victimized, Mrs. Papastavrou had struck back. Every evening since her removal upstairs, she appeared on the balcony on the dot of half past six and moaned loudly until seven o'clock. Sometimes, when the weather was particularly warm, she gave a matinée performance. Often, well-meaning passers-by called ambulances, but she was returned almost immediately.

Binny looked out of the window to make certain the old woman remained indoors, and was appalled at the amount of refuse lying about the path. There were even eggshells caught in the branches of the privet hedge. "Ought I to sweep it up?" she asked aloud.

A tub, placed on bricks, stood in front of the row of dust bins. In it was planted some sort of bush that never did anything. It had been meant to act as a screen. The bin lids had been stolen long ago. A fat dog from up the street kept waddling in and tipping out the garbage.

"Sweep what?" said Lucy.

"The front path. It's a sight."

"Why not?" said Lucy. "You could dust the weeds while you're at it." She rolled off the sofa and lay face downwards, drumming on the floor with her toe-caps.

Even though it would be dark when the Simpsons arrived, the headlamps of their car would light up the square of garden laid with crazy paving. Mrs. Simpson would see the rubbish clearly illuminated.

Below the window was a strip of earth dangerously littered with strands of barbed wire, intended to discourage cats from doing their business on the stunted daffodils. Wrought-iron railings ran from the side of the front door, along the flower border, and ended at the steps to the basement flat. The basement was owned by a young couple, though Edward, in Binny's presence, had once told a colleague that it was hers and she rented it out. Anxious to boast of her assets, he referred to the young couple as her tenants.

Several betting slips, flung down by disappointed racing men, whirled upward from the path and, catching on the barbed wire, fluttered like sandwich flags among the daffodils.

I can do no more, thought Binny, rubbing at the window pane with a duster. She could hardly be blamed for the untidy habits of dogs and gamblers. And even supposing Mrs. Simpson noticed the mess, it wasn't likely she'd rush in muttering her complaints before she'd had a chance to be introduced.

Pushing the matter from her mind, Binny moved from the window and, tripping over her daughter's body, ran headlong into the kitchen.

Lucy rose and went upstairs to fetch Alison. Binny knelt on hands and knees and picked up tobacco grains from the floor.

A low keening began outside in the street. Hands clutching the rail, clouds scudding above her bowed head, Mrs. Papastavrou swayed backwards and forwards.

It was as well, thought Binny, that the Simpsons weren't coming until eight o'clock. Edward pretended that he didn't mind about Mrs. Papastavrou, that he'd grown used to her. But he hadn't. He stood well back from the window, both saddened and embarrassed, while the children snickered with laughter and the old lady, marooned on her balcony, wailed like a banshee.

"Alison won't," said Lucy, coming back into the room.

"Well, make her," shouted Binny, stamping her foot. She was beginning to breathe quite heavily. "I would be grateful if you would get your own things together as well. Have you got your night-dress?"

"Don't be bloody wet," said Lucy. She went to the table and tore at a French loaf with her teeth.

"I don't want to remind you of the shirt I bought you," Binny said. "Or the pair of shoes costing twenty-four pounds that you said you couldn't live without and promptly gave to your friend Soggy. When I was your age I was grateful if my mother gave me a smile."

"I lent them, you fool," corrected Lucy.

Binny's voice became shrill. "I've long since given up expecting gratitude or common courtesy, but I do expect you to get Alison and yourself out of the house. It's little enough to ask, God knows."

"Keep your lid on," said Lucy. She began to comb her hair at the mirror. Strands of hair and crumbs of bread fell to the hearth. Binny could feel a pulse beating in her throat. She burned with fury. No wonder she never put on an ounce of weight. The daily aggravation the children caused her was probably comparable to a five-mile run or an hour with the skipping rope. Clutching the region of her heart and fighting for self-control, she said insincerely, "Darling, you can be very sensitive and persuasive. Just tell her Sybil's waiting and that there's ice cream and things."

Lucy strolled into the hall and called loudly, "Come down, Alison, or I'll bash your teeth in."

After several minutes a sound of barking was heard on the first-floor landing.

"Baby," crooned Binny, going upstairs with outstretched arms. Alison was on all fours, crouched against the wall. Binny often told friends it was nothing to worry about. Until two years ago Alison had insisted on baring her tummy button in the street and rubbing it against lamp posts. She had grown out of that, as doubtless she would soon grow tired of pretending she was a dog.

"Come along, darling," said Binny brightly. She bent down and patted her daughter's head.

Alison growled and seized Binny's ankle in her teeth.

Putting both hands behind her to resist hitting the child, Binny descended the stairs.

Lucy was at the sink pouring cooking sherry into a milk bottle.

"Out, out, out," cried Binny. "I am not here to provide booze for your layabout friends. This is not an off-licence."

She frogmarched Lucy to the door and pushed her down the steps. Alison began to cry. Running down the path, Binny caught up with Lucy at the hedge and put desperate arms about her. She said urgently, "Now please, pull yourself together. Get your things, take your coat, and I'll give you a pound note to spend."

Smirking, Lucy re-entered the house and began to put on her flying jacket. Smothering her youngest daughter in kisses, Binny took her to the door. She nodded blindly as Alison climbed the fence.

"You're crying, Mummy," called Alison. Her mouth quivered.

"I'm very happy, darling," said Binny. "Don't you worry about me." She wiped her cheeks with her hand. "I'm going to have a lovely party." She stood there waving until Alison was let into the Evans'.

Lucy had locked herself in the bathroom. Binny blew crumbs off the tablecloth and attended to the cushions on the sofa. She cut the end off the mutilated loaf and straightened the reproduction of The Last Supper that hung askew on the wall. Then she called gently down the hall that she would like to use the lavatory.

"Go away," snarled Lucy. "I'm trying to have a crap."

Binny left a pound note on the table and climbed the stairs. She walked round and round her bedroom humming fiercely. At that moment she fully understood Mrs. Papastavrou, fluttering in the wind and protesting for all the world to hear.

After a time Lucy shouted that she was off now. Binny kept silent.

"Well, come on. Give us a kiss."

"I certainly won't," called Binny. "You're far too rude."

The door slammed violently. Instantly remorseful, Binny ran to the window and watched her daughter walk sullenly along the gutter. She looked such a little girl, aggressively scuffing the ground with the studs of her massive boots. At the same age Binny had been married and looking after a house. She rapped frantically on the pane of glass; she blew kisses. Lucy disappeared round the corner.

Binny turned and banged her hip painfully against the edge of the ping-pong table. Every week she meant to advertise it for sale in the local newspaper. It had been brought three years ago for the children; she had hoped it might keep them off the streets. Selflessly she had moved her bed and her wardrobe into the back half of the room so that there would be somewhere to put it. After six weeks of their constant bickering, turfing her personal belongings ruthlessly onto the landing to make additional space, and bringing their friends in at all hours of the day and night, sometimes even when Binny was asleep, she had forbidden them the use of the room. They didn't seem to grasp how irritating it was for her to lie there with her face-cream on and be subjected to large unknown youths clambering under and over her bed in the pursuit of ping-pong balls. She couldn't think where they learned such behavior, though she suspected it was being taught in the schools. They couldn't spell and they didn't read and they had little respect for property. Like a vast army on the move they swarmed across the city playing gramophone records and frequenting public houses. It wasn't that they disliked adults—they simply didn't notice them. Devoted to their homes, it was obvious that they would never leave. The only edge they had on an earlier generation was their casual regard for animals; they didn't pull wings off flies or throw stones at cats.

Rubbing her side, Binny was about to take off her coat when she heard a knock at the front door. Alarmed, she crept onto the landing. It could be any one of a number of people, none of them welcome—Alison deceived over the ice cream and returning in tears, the woman from No. 52 looking for her cat, the arrears collector from the television rental service? It was too early surely for the Simpsons to have arrived.

Thinking it might be Lucy come back for a

cuddle, she went hopefully downstairs and opened the door.

"Are you the cleaning woman?" A stout black man advanced into the hall. His neck was encased in plaster of Paris.

"No," said Binny.

"I am bringing a message for you and all believing strangers, so that you may have a chance of redemption."

"I don't really think I'm a believer," Binny said.

"The eyes of the Lord are over the righteous," claimed the man, taking no notice. His own eyes were fixed on a point directly above Binny's left shoulder. "His ears are open to their prayers, but the face of the Lord is against them that do evil. And who is he that will harm you if you be followers of that which is good?"

"I'm rather busy at the moment," said Binny.

"All that He asks is that you should follow Him."

"Still," protested Binny, "I haven't much time."

She was relieved to see Edward stepping out of a taxi at the curb, holding several bottles in his arms.

"Luke xv:7," preached the black man relentlessly. "Who are the just persons who need no repentance?" He was watching the stairs, as if waiting for somebody to appear.

Edward came up the path. Binny thought he

looked terribly attractive. She usually thought that when he came towards her unexpectedly; later it wore off. Lucy addressed him as "Fatso" whenever she saw him; but really, in his dark City suit and his shirt with the pale stripe, he seemed very trim and dapper. He reminded Binny of a pre-war father come home ready for his Ovaltine —pipe in mouth, the evening newspaper under his arm. She did find him attractive, but when he went on about his roses or blew his nose like a trumpet or fell over when he stood on one trembling leg to remove his sock, she was at a loss to understand why.

"Are you going somewhere?" he demanded. "It's gone seven, you know."

"This gentleman's from the Bible," said Binny. "We were just having a little chat."

"Well, I should hurry it up if I were you." Edward pushed past them and went into the kitchen.

"Now that your man's home," the black man decided, "I'd best be going. He'll want his tea." He told her he'd leave a copy of his magazine and she ought to look at the questions at the back. Possibly when he called next week she'd have answered a few of them.

"I shouldn't count on it," said Binny, stung at the speed with which he was prepared to be on his way now that "her" man had returned. He hadn't minded wasting her time; it hadn't occurred to him that she too might have been wanting her tea.

Edward poured her out a drink before she went upstairs to do her face. He congratulated her on the table—he admired the flowers in the center. He forbore to mention that the vase could do with a wash.

"Food smells good," he said, anxious to be appreciative.

"There's nothing cooking yet," she said. "It isn't time."

He sat her on his lap and, relinquishing his pipe, kissed her. She couldn't respond wholeheartedly because of her headscarf. She felt faded and work-worn.

He said huskily. "Are the children gone?"

She nodded.

"Can't we go upstairs?"

"No," she said. "I'm not in the mood. Lucy was awful."

"I've had the devil of a day," said Edward. "One thing after another."

"She made Alison cry."

"The telephone never stopped ringing."

"I feel odd," she confided. "That man telling me there was nothing to fear—and earlier on when I was out shopping people kept waving."

Edward attempted to push his hand inside the front of her coat but it was tightly buttoned.

"Why *my* door?" she asked.

"*I'd* knock on your door," Edward said urgently. "Any time."

"You've been drinking," said Binny. She suddenly remembered the taxi drawing into the curb and felt resentful. He never came in his car in case somebody recognized the number plate and told his wife. "I can't imagine why you think you've had the devil of a day. What with your eight-course lunches and visits to the pub—"

"Three," he corrected.

"Nobody cooked *my* lunch. And look at the way that man ran off because he thought it was time for your tea. Talk about the chosen people of this world—"

"He didn't look chosen to me," said Edward. "Somebody obviously tried to break his neck."

He wanted Binny to get into the bath so that he could scrub her back. She said she'd already bathed, and he said why didn't he get in the bath then and she could wash his back.

"I'm not having you wallowing and snorting in my clean bath," she told him, and went upstairs to take off her coat and scarf.

She stood in the cramped bedroom and combed her hair. She felt crushed, flattened in some way. It was Edward's fault, coming in a taxi like that and not wanting to know about Lucy being rude. He always slid away when she mentioned the children. Of course, his own son was too busy learning Latin and Greek and generally behaving like Little Lord Fauntleroy to cause him a moment's trouble. Why, she wondered, was Edward always trying to get her into soapy water? It must have some connection with his days at boarding school; he probably thought it more hygienic to do it in the bath.

She didn't know why she felt so despairing inside. All the big issues were over and done with —it wasn't likely now that she'd get pregnant and even if she did, nobody, not even her mother, was going to tell her off. She didn't have any financial problems, she didn't hanker after new carpets. She didn't hanker after anything—certainly not Edward with a block of soap in one hand and that pipe spilling ash down her spine.

She was compelled suddenly to stand very still. She felt like an animal in long grass scenting smoke on the wind. She saw her reflection in the dressing-table mirror; she was holding a green comb to her head and staring fixedly at the glass. It had been the same this morning when she was out with Alma; only then there had been so much noise, so many faces with insinuating smiles— voices calling her name. Was it because she'd sent Lucy away without kissing her? Was Gregory lying battered by football hooligans on the floor of a tube train to Clapham? With the children gone, the whole house was heavy with silence.

It was Edward, she decided, who was upsetting her. He lived too much in the past; all that rubbish about his dormitory and the shadows on the playing fields. He evaded her completely. He should be dragged, by that schoolboy lock of hair falling over one nostalgic eye, into the present. She was fed up with his fumblings on the sofa, as if it was still those days before the war when mothers kept coming in and out with trays of tea and courting was a furtive thing. Why couldn't he pretend that he longed to leave his wife, so that she in return could pretend she wished he would? He ought to forget the ins and outs of capital transfer tax, and the particular type of pest that plagued his fruit bushes, and discuss what he did with Helen at night when she'd come back from all those meetings. They could have a row over it and be moved to tears, and then they both might feel something, some emotion that would nudge them closer to one another. Obviously he did do something with Helen. He was far too uncomplicated a man to abstain when there was a body lying next to him in bed, and apart from his roses it wasn't as if he had any hobbies to take his mind off sex. Old Simpson was quite right to disapprove of his carryings on. What Edward should do, she told herself, as though discussing somebody she had never met, was to park his car actually outside the house. In full view. After he made love he should lie there dozing and not trot into the darkness desperate for a taxi. Though he removed his socks and even put down his pipe during the act, he could not bring himself to unbuckle the watch from his wrist. Sometimes, when he lay exhausted on top of Binny, a little to one side with his cheek resting on his arm, she knew he was looking squint-eyed at the time.

She put away her comb and brushed the shoulders of her dress. That was the worst of black, it showed the slightest speck of dust; by the time she'd cooked the dinner she'd be spotted with grease. Except for the end of that French loaf, Lucy probably wouldn't have a bite of food until tomorrow morning. It was madness putting complete strangers before one's own flesh and blood. She had enough to do fighting hormone losses and hot flushes and depressions that dropped out of nowhere, without being tormented by guilt.

Belligerently she flung down the clothes-brush and returned to Edward, who was seated at the table with the evening newspaper spread before him.

"I think I should start cooking," she said. "Don't you?"

"Yes," he agreed. It was, he realized, ten minutes to eight. "Can I help?"

But he didn't move. He and Binny had another glass of wine.

She was sure the Simpsons were late. She kept asking the time, but Edward answered casually, saying, "What? Oh, the time . . . Jolly early if you ask me." It wouldn't do to get her into a state.

After half an hour Binny said the chops were ruined. Greatly alarmed, he rose to his feet.

"Well, almost," she amended. "What shall I do with them?"

He didn't know what to advise. Helen produced perfectly edible meals in an effortless way, and he was a bit thrown by the atmosphere of panic generated by Binny at the stove.

"Well, look at them," Binny shouted, bringing the grilling tray to the table and thrusting the chops under his nose.

They were a little wizened, he thought, but otherwise normal. "They're lovely," he said. "Simply lovely."

"Don't you ever do any cooking?" she asked. There was a hostile note in her voice.

He bent over the crossword and prayed the Simpsons would arrive soon.

Some minutes later Binny demanded to know if he did any washing.

"Washing?" he queried, playing for time.

"Do you wash your smalls?"

"We've a washing machine," he said.

"Even for your smalls?"

"It's for everything," he said. "Big or small."

She wanted him to describe his washing arrangements in detail.

It seemed a funny thing to be interested in. "Well," he said. "I put my clothing, underpants, socks and so forth, in a polythene bag in the bathroom and Helen places them, in due course, in the machine."

"And you let her?" Binny cried, as though they were discussing coal-heaving or some equally strenuous job.

Inwardly he grew rattled. It was unfair of Binny to attack him over his underpants just because the Simpsons were late and she was worried about the chops. "Look here," he protested, "I have enough to do in the office, you know, without worrying about the washing. Helen's in all day. It's no trouble if you've got a machine. Besides, I don't know how to load the thing. As a matter of fact she won't let me touch it. It's her department."

"Do you sleep with her?"

The question was so unexpected that his mouth fell open. He felt he'd suffered a minor stroke. "My love," he began inadequately.

"You do, don't you?"

"No, no," he protested. He knew she knew he was not telling the truth. "She's not one for that sort of thing," he floundered. "Not now. She's gone off it."

Binny abandoned her place at the stove and came to sit at the table. She smiled lovingly at him.

He said uneasily, "I do care for you, you know. I really do."

"We all go off it," said Binny. "Us women." She held her fourth glass of wine to her lips and drank. "Until somebody exciting comes along. Like you," she added generously and, reaching out, attempted to touch his cheek.

He ducked, thinking she was going to strike him.

"Take Helen," she continued. "She's used to you. You're the old sod that's part of the furniture."

It wasn't, he felt, a flattering description. Still, Binny was smiling in an affectionate manner. He allowed her, without flinching, to caress his face.

"You're not a mystery any more," she told him. "Probably if you stayed very still she'd run a duster over you. But if a bloke came along, someone she'd never set eyes on, well . . . stands to reason, doesn't it?"

"Does it?" he said.

Binny withdrew her hand and thumped the table. "I bet you if the milkman rushed in and grabbed old Helen, she wouldn't say no."

"Perhaps not," he said dubiously. He had a mental picture of his wife moving serenely about the kitchen in her housecoat, and the youth from United Dairies running through the door in his striped apron and flinging her to the floor. "Of course," he said. "There's always the possibility that she might phone the police instead."

Outside it had grown dark. The block of flats across the street was transformed into a glittering mass of glass and concrete. Behind net curtains shadowed with the leaves of rubber plants, blurred figures moved across rooms that blazed with light.

"Six letters," said Edward, looking down at his paper. "Beginning with T."

"Terror," said Binny.

"A hard case," said Edward. "Turtle." And he pencilled it in.

5

Driving in their car across London, the Simpsons exchanged bitter words. Outwardly it was on account of Muriel's interpretation of the street map of N.W.6. They took a left turning instead of a right and ended up on the wrong side of the park.

"Well, go through the park then," advised Muriel, but in fact the gates were locked. They made a minor detour, during which Simpson hunched his shoulders meanly and swore several times.

"Why are you behaving like a fool?" she asked.

"You never see anything clearly," he accused. "You haven't the wit."

"I try," she murmured, thinking he was referring to her map reading. "I don't have X-ray vision. I did tell you to stop under a lamp."

"God knows what we're getting mixed up in," shouted Simpson. "We don't know this woman from Adam."

Muriel pointed out reasonably that they didn't know a lot of people. Why, only last week they'd had dinner with a young couple neither of them had met before. It had been an enjoyable occasion, even if he'd complained afterwards that the main course was stone cold. "Though I can't think how you noticed," she said. "You were so busy ogling the girl." Muriel hadn't been perturbed by his behavior. She knew her husband acted as if he had a roving eye, but really he was seeking attention, not giving it. To her knowledge he was a puritan and an egotist. She considered him incapable of indulging in more than a wink and a nudge; it might interfere with his golf.

"Last week," Simpson reminded her heatedly, "was business. Bloody bread-and-butter business. The sort of thing that pays the bills and puts the clothes on your back."

He was thinking how unfair it was that the nicer moments of life—a few drinks under the belt, good food, a pretty woman seated opposite— were invariably spent in the company of one's wife.

"Of course," he said, "I know you don't give a damn about that, as long as you manage to get out of the house and have another excuse for going to the hairdressers, but there are one or two mundane things that have to be paid for." He proceeded to list a few of them—the mortgage, the tax on her car, the red telephones she'd insisted on installing. He ended by telling her that Edward Freeman was in a potentially dangerous situation; didn't she realize it could lead to blackmail?

"Don't be absurd," said Muriel. "He's not a member of the Cabinet. Besides, what has it to do with my telephones? It's no good shouting at me. He's your friend, not mine. I had nothing to do with the arrangements. As for getting out of the house, I'm perfectly capable of opening a door. I have merely to turn the handle."

"Go to bloody hell," ordered Simpson.

He almost took the wrong turning at the next roundabout. Muriel remained silent but pointed a contemptuous finger, at the last moment, in the correct direction.

It was raining heavily as they drove into Fulton Street. Simpson cruised slowly past a row of terraced houses, a block of flats, a further line of houses in a dilapidated condition, and a garage. Reaching the end of the road he reversed some distance down an alley and drove back the way they had come.

"Aren't the trees pretty?" said Muriel. "The raindrops look like flakes of snow." She smiled.

Simpson stopped the car. He sat there with his leather gloves resting on the wheel and his plump thighs splayed wide. "I've forgotten the number," he confessed. "Freeman said something about a black-and-white cat, and some sort of creeper hanging over the balcony."

"Knock on doors," suggested Muriel. "Look at the names under the bell."

She watched him sprinting across the road with the rain falling on him. She knew he didn't remember the name either.

He ran up and down steps, peering at windows and glancing now and then at the car. She waved encouragingly once or twice. After a while he returned and slumped damply into the driving seat.

"No luck," said Muriel. There was a funny smell coming from his suede overcoat.

"I've got it," cried Simpson. "His car. Freeman's car. It's a brown Rover. It'll be outside the house." He turned the key in the ignition.

"He won't have come by car," said Muriel. "Just drive very slowly and we'll look for vegetation."

There were three balconies, next to each other, entwined with thin strands of creeper. On Muriel's instructions Simpson went up the steps of the second house and knocked on the door. Here the vine, coming into bud, hung low and dripped water down his neck. Muriel remained in the warmth of the car. The house was in complete darkness.

Edward plucked Simpson inside with such haste that to Muriel, observing the scene from behind a window distorted by rain, it was as if her husband had simply been swallowed up. She stared curiously at the empty porch.

Simpson's propulsion into the hall was painful; he was pierced in the ankle by a sharp implement. His small cry of agony went unnoticed amid the enthusiasm of his welcome.

To Edward, the arrival of Simpson was comparable to sighting the cavalry on the brow of the hill when all seemed lost. He hit his friend repeatedly on the shoulder as though they'd not met in years.

"My wife," said Simpson. "She's still out there." He tore himself from Edward's embrace and hobbled down the steps.

"What on earth happened to you?" asked Muriel. "Why are you being so silly?"

"I was stabbed," said Simpson, gritting his teeth and locking the car.

Muriel took no notice. He was always complaining of aches and pains; he had no stamina. She stood on the pavement in the rain, trying to protect her hair with her arms. The privet hedge, she noted, illuminated by the block of flats across the street, was festooned with egg shells, strewn among the dripping leaves like Christmas baubles on a tree.

"Aren't they stopping after all?" asked Binny, confused by the comings and goings. She stood at the table, rearranging the flowers in the white vase.

"They're on their way," said Edward. "Simpson forgot his wife. He's gone to fetch her." And he ran out again to wait for them behind the door.

Simpson, followed by Muriel, re-entered the house with caution. In the gloom he saw the outline of a bicycle leaning against the wall.

"Such weather," murmured Muriel, peering downwards for somewhere to wipe her feet.

Edward led them into the front room. "This is George Simpson," he said, speaking to Binny.

Simpson saw a small woman with a pale face, dressed in mourning. She was holding a pink carnation in her hand.

"And his wife, Miriam—"

"Muriel," corrected Simpson. He bent and rubbed at his ankle. He felt sure he was bleeding.

"We weren't certain of the house," Muriel said. "It was in darkness."

"Edward made me draw the shutters," explained Binny. "He doesn't like being overlooked."

"It's cosier, don't you think?" cried Edward. "Keeps the place warm. I felt rather chilly myself, though I did turn up the thermostat." He looked anxiously at Muriel, fearing he'd sounded too familiar with the central heating system.

Simpson said shutters were splendid. It was just like France. So much better than curtains.

They all gazed at the windows and nodded in agreement. The metal bar that kept the shutters in place, once fixed, was difficult to unclasp. The

64

children, impatient to let in daylight at breakfast-time, were in the habit of jabbing at the bar with a poker to release it; most of the paintwork and portions of the wood panelling were severely damaged.

"We did have curtains," said Binny. "But they fell down." She knew Edward was observing her critically—watching her face, her movements, noticing the way she spoke. Often, when she felt particularly rested and well, he would tell her she looked tired.

"I'd better take that upstairs," she said, admiring the expensive fur about Muriel's shoulders. She would have taken Simpson's coat too, but he kept bending down and fiddling with his sock.

"Please don't trouble," Muriel said, looking round for somewhere safe to lodge the cape. "Any old place will do."

But Binny insisted. When she held the fur in her arms it felt like some animal drowned in a pond. She ran upstairs stroking it tenderly, and laid it across the ping-pong table.

Simpson remembered he'd left a bottle of wine in the car. He would fetch it at once.

"Don't bother, old boy," said Edward. "We've plenty to drink, believe you me."

"Nonsense," Simpson said. "I won't be a jiffy."

Limping painfully down the steps, he turned left at the hedge and began to run as fast as his injured ankle would allow, along the street in the direction of the garage. Earlier, when he'd been looking for the house, he'd observed a telephone box through the rear window of the car. Stumbling down the alleyway, he saw a man running from the opposite end of the lane towards him. They reached the kiosk at the same time.

"Do you mind?" said the man. "I've a taxi waiting. The wife's just had a baby." He pulled open the door and went inside.

Simpson fumed. He had tried unsuccessfully all afternoon to make a telephone call. When Muriel was in the bedroom dressing for dinner he'd tried again, but just as he was getting through he'd thought he heard her on the stairs. He strolled up and down, struggling for breath. There was a taxi with its engine running parked in the main street at the end of the alley.

He heard the man say, "Yes . . . no complications . . . about half an hour ago." When he came out of the box he was smiling.

"Congratulations," Simpson said grudgingly.

"Ta," said the man.

Simpson dialled the number. "Hello . . . is that Marcia?"

"No, it isn't, I'm afraid," said a masculine voice. "Hold on, I'll get her."

Marcia came to the phone and asked who it was.

"It's me . . . George. Was that the candidate fellow I just spoke to?"

"He's out," she said.

"Oh. It was Lloyd, was it?"

"No it wasn't, sweetie. Just a friend. Why are you ringing?"

"We were out for dinner and I thought I'd say Hello." He'd always impressed on Marcia that he wasn't the sort of chap to run around behind his wife's back. That wasn't his style at all. He and his wife, he had told her, went their own separate ways. Within certain limits, he was a free agent. "We're in a very nice house in the Park," he said.

"With a call box?"

"There's an office in the house. The fellow's a merchant banker. I wondered if you're free to-morrow night?"

"Oh, sweetie . . . what a shame. I'm not."

"Well, what about lunch then?"

He thought he heard someone whispering at the other end of the line.

"Look here, sweetie," Marcia said. "Give me a tinkle at the office in the morning. I'll let you know then."

"All right," he said.

Hobbling, he scurried back up the road.

Edward gave the guests a little sherry to sip before dinner. He didn't offer any to Binny. The Simpsons wanted to sit on the sofa, but Edward forestalled them. "It's a shade uncomfortable," he said, and laughed. He had made love to Binny many times on the sofa, though it was too short for him to lie full length upon it. His left knee, exposed to constant friction on the hair-cord covering of the floor, was permanently scarred.

When he was in the car sometimes, driving to work, or in the office talking to a client, he would gently touch this proof of passion with his fingertips and wince with happiness. He was ready, should Helen notice the wound, to tell her he feared he was becoming increasingly knock-kneed as the years advanced.

"I do admire those cushions," Muriel said. She would have liked to go somewhere and attend to her wet hair.

"Have one," said Binny. "Have one." And she placed a cushion on a chair at the table and told everybody to sit down. She couldn't concentrate on the cooking with the Simpsons standing about looking uncomfortable. Edward opened a bottle of wine.

The guests perched on the damaged chairs and put their elbows on the table to steady themselves.

Muriel frowned at her husband. He was bent sideways, dragging the cloth with his stomach, doing something out of sight. "The traffic," she said. "It was simply chaotic. We thought we'd never get here, didn't we, George?"

"Don't tell me," protested Edward. He walked backward and forward in front of the mirror, holding a glass in his hand.

"No trouble with parking though," said Simpson. "Not here at any rate."

"Never any trouble here," Edward agreed.

"You don't do any parking here," said Binny.

6

They began dinner at a quarter past nine. Edward wondered agitatedly how he could possibly manage to eat, help with the washing up, and be out of the house by half-past ten at the latest. It would seem fearfully abrupt.

There was grapefruit to start with.

"Excellent, excellent," Simpson said, gouging the fruit from its skin with a spoon that had buckled, without warning, in his hand.

"The reason the loaf looks funny," explained Binny, "is because one of my children was hungry." Her voice quivered slightly. Recovering, she handed the sugar bowl to Muriel. "You've got four, haven't you? All boys. Edward told me."

"Two, actually," interrupted Simpson.

"Two girls," Muriel said. "We're quite pleased with them. Of course, I never went out to work or anything like that, and I didn't have a nanny when they were younger. I think it's important to give them one's undivided attention, don't you? And I'm glad now that I had them all to myself."

"I'm glad I didn't have a weapon in the house," said Binny. "I'd have murdered mine years ago."

"My father," Edward told them, "had a nanny who hanged herself."

"No," screamed Muriel.

"Yes, she did. It's as true as I'm sitting here. My father was grown up of course, but he heard about it. It seemed her mind snapped under the strain. One by one, losing her babies in the mud. Master Charles, Master Guy—"

"In the mud?" said Binny. "Are you sure?"

"The trenches," explained Simpson. "In France." He shook his head somberly from side to side.

Anxious to change the subject, Muriel confided that her daughters were musically inclined; she hinted that they were fairly competent on the recorder.

"My girls have frightful voices," said Binny, thinking of tape machines. "And their language—" Her eyes filled with tears.

She put down her spoon and stared distressed at a segment of grapefruit on her plate. Nobody noticed. Edward was telling the Simpsons that houses like these were a jolly sensible investment.

Gilt-edged in fact. With inflation and so forth, and the cutting back of the government building program, superior properties in London would eventually be unobtainable. "We've seen the end of the downward spiral in prices," he said. "The slump is over."

"How many floors are there?" asked Simpson. The house didn't seem particularly superior, what little he could see of it. He wondered if the place was divided into flats. There was certainly something wrong with the electricity supply; the room was full of shadows. He sought with his foot for the table leg and gently worked at removing his shoe.

"Three," said Edward.

"Four with the basement," Binny said. "I've let it at the moment." She tried not to look at Simpson. Edward had told her that Simpson's little sortie to the V.D. clinic was to do with some woman he'd met in the bar at a theater. She'd written her telephone number on his program when his wife had slipped off to the Ladies. Edward said Simpson had given good money for getting his leg over, because that way his lapse would be more likely to be understood, should he be caught out. Binny hadn't been able to understand it. Neither she nor any of her friends had ever been paid for doing it. She'd thought at the time that Simpson had made the whole thing up out of his head; he was boasting. Now she wasn't so sure.

"My dear girl," cried Edward. He rapped boisterously on his plate with a spoon. "Who's telling a little white lie?" He turned to Muriel and explained that Binny's ex-husband had sold off the basement several years ago to meet various business commitments. As he spoke he regretted that he'd addressed Binny as his dear girl; Simpson had warned him about hanky panky. "Mind you," he said, "the basement isn't really much of an asset. It's a little dark and there's no garden to speak of at the back. No garden at all, actually. We've got quite a large garden—fruit trees, roses, one or two vegetables. I do a little potting in the greenhouse . . . take a few cuttings . . . nothing special. Are you a gardener, Miriam?"

"Muriel," said Simpson.

Confused, Edward poured out more wine. He said loudly, "Helen's not too keen on the spade work, but she likes it in summer—tea on the lawn, that sort of caper."

Binny rose abruptly and took the saucers to the sink.

"Get up, George," ordered Muriel. "Take things into the kitchen." She herself, seeing Edward was puffing at his pipe, took a cigarette from her handbag and lit it.

Simpson carried the sugar bowl and spoons through to Binny. As she stood there at the stove, the top of her tongue protruding as she concentrated on arranging chops and grilled tomatoes on a large blue plate, he thought how young she looked. Of course he knew the lighting was poor and she was no chicken, but the droop of her narrow shoulders and the little curls falling about her neck enchanted him. Muriel was tall with wide shoulders and strong as an ox. She had on two occasions moved their upright piano single-handed from one wall to another. He had refused to help, on the grounds that he might strain his back. He didn't want to mark the parquet floor and he never dreamt she could do it alone. Putting her firm buttocks against the back of the heavy instrument and bending at the knees like Groucho Marx, she had shoved it clear across the room.

"You mustn't lift that," he said, stricken, as Binny gripped the blue plate in both hands. He took it from her, thinking she was far too fragile to carry such a load.

Edward was speaking in low tones to Muriel. He champed on the stem of his pipe and nodded his head emphatically. Binny, bringing the roast potatoes to the table, imagined he was saying that there was nothing between them, that he just felt sorry for her.

At the arrival of the meat, Edward jumped to his feet and removed his jacket. He flung it carelessly on the sofa. A comb and a fountain pen slid from his pocket and fell to the carpet. Because of his belly, which was large, he was obliged to wear braces to keep up his trousers. Finding the elastic too uncomfortable on his shoulders, he jerked the braces free and let them dangle about his thighs.

'What on earth are you doing?' said Binny. He looked a sight, with his rumpled shirt and those striped lengths of elastic hanging like two large catapults from his waist.

"It's damned hot in here," he said, forgetting that earlier he had used the coldness of the room as an excuse to close the shutters. He scooped up his belongings from the floor, lost his balance, and careered against the table. Spluttering with laughter and red in the face, he collapsed heavily on to his chair. "Aren't there any greens?" he asked.

"Salad only," Binny told him.

"Rabbit fodder," he said sadly, and undid the top button of his shirt.

Simpson couldn't help admiring the man. He was definitely an eccentric. Of course he could afford to be, on his salary, but still. He asked if anybody minded if he too removed his coat.

"Do as you please," said Muriel. She found the food plentiful and well cooked; the salad had the right amount of garlic in the dressing and the roast potatoes were crisp. It was obvious to her that Edward Freeman was in no danger from Binny. It was just the reverse. *He* was evidently using *her*. Some women liked that sort of thing, she knew. Binny was the right size and weight to be submissive; perhaps she had a father complex and liked some big rough man treating her in a patronizing fashion and ticking her off about the vegetables. She wouldn't be at all surprised if Edward didn't slap her now and then.

He, for his part, found Muriel very pleasant to talk to. Simpson must have been over-reacting when he'd implied she might be standoffish this evening. After all, any woman who had been involved in that X, Y and Z business must be jolly approachable; he couldn't imagine anyone asking Helen if they could borrow the spare room. Muriel cared about gardening too, he could tell. She wasn't lyrical over it, but she seemed knowledgeable about insecticides.

"Of course, I was brought up in the country," he said. "So I suppose it's in the blood. This feeling for the land. My father inherited an estate in Norfolk and I learned early to have a healthy respect for the soil. Just a small estate," he added hastily, hoping Binny hadn't overheard. Whenever he'd mentioned his father's property before, she'd doffed an imaginary cap and talked about tugging his forelock. "My earliest memories," he told Simpson's wife, "are of being woken by father at dawn, and going out with the guns to shoot."

"How lovely," murmured Muriel.

"I had to stand up to my waist in icy water for hours, waiting for the duck to fly. Couldn't have been more than eight or nine years of age."

"How ghastly," said Muriel.

"You've no idea what pleasure it gives me to see Helen in the garden, sitting in the deckchair by the fence, shelling peas that I've grown myself.

It's the sense of achievement. Nothing like it. Have some more wine."

Muriel said thank you and held out her glass for him to fill.

She was a pretty woman, he realized, and fond of her food. She wore the right clothes; pale blue was a favorite color of his. He looked across at Binny. She was wearing a severe black dress that personally he thought dowdy. She had little broken veins on her cheeks and chest. He couldn't see them without his reading glasses but he knew they were there. When she got up from the table, as she did frequently, to fetch butter knives and salt, she waddled.

"Does George do much in the garden?" Edward asked.

"No," said Muriel. "Not much. He works late most nights, and then he has trouble with his back."

One day, thought Edward gloomily, Simpson was going to be caught out. They were all going to be caught out—Simpson, himself, those other foolish men drinking in public houses, jingling the loose change in their pockets and boasting of affairs. It was astonishing how fashionable it was to be unfaithful. He often wondered if it had anything to do with going without a hat. No sooner had the homburgs and the bowlers disappeared from the City than everyone grew their hair longer, and after that nothing was sacred.

Flushed with the wine and wanting to make

amends to someone, Edward leaned towards Muriel and said softly: "You got me out of a hole, you know. I'm very grateful."

Muriel didn't quite catch what he'd said. She thought perhaps he was offering her another drink. "No," she protested. "I can't take any more." She raised her hand and made a little gesture of refusal that Edward found charming.

"Seriously," he murmured, twisting round in his chair so that Binny wouldn't hear, "I can't tell you, Miriam, how much I appreciate it. She's a wonderful girl, but in the past she's sneered at people. People I've mentioned. You know . . . friends of mine. She says I don't know any people, not real people, not ones with flesh and blood—"

"Yes, of course," agreed Muriel.

"When she says 'blood,' she sort of curls her lip back . . . over her teeth . . . like a vampire." Here Edward gave a facial imitation of Binny in one of her more contemptuous moments. "See what I mean?" he said.

Muriel noticed that he had a fragment of watercress lodged in his teeth at the side. "I think I saw it on television," she said, but he was leaning back in his chair and watching Simpson.

How lucky, thought Edward, to have such friends. Look at the way Simpson was putting himself out to be nice to Binny—cracking jokes, taking off his jacket, talking to her quite naturally. Perhaps there was some way round that business of the office cleaning expenses. He knew Simpson probably thought Binny a bit of an oddity. He'd met Simpson's latest woman—she was tall and brisk and called Simpson "sweetie." She had a flat somewhere off the Kilburn High Road, which she shared with two men, one of whom was a Liberal party candidate. Though it wasn't likely that Helen would know him, it was a bit of a shock when he'd first heard about it. He inclined his head and listened to what Simpson was saying.

". . . so she went to the surgery first thing in the morning and she said, Doctor, Doctor, is there something radically wrong? Whenever my husband makes love to me, he puts his ear to my chest and hears music. Unbutton your blouse, my good woman—"

"Good Lord," cried Edward, greatly excited. "I heard that joke only this morning."

"Perhaps you should tell it then," said Simpson.

"It's jolly good," Edward told Muriel. "I'm not sure how it ends, but this woman goes to the doctor because she—"

"I've lost the pudding," said Binny. She rose from the table and went into the kitchen to look inside the cupboard.

"Won't it be in the oven?" asked Edward. He shambled after her, holding his trousers up with his hands.

"I didn't put it in the oven," said Binny.

Edward called loudly, "She's lost the pudding," but Muriel was standing beside her husband with her hand resting on his shoulder. They both appeared to be discussing the picture of The Last Supper that hung on the wall.

"Have you looked properly?" Edward said. He bent down and peered inside the oven.

"It doesn't matter," said Binny. She squatted beside him and whispered, "I thought you said he was an ass. I think he's attractive."

"Is he?" Edward was surprised. Simpson was small and swarthy and he was losing his hair. "Well, I'm no judge of that," he said bleakly, and managed to smile. He was consumed with jealousy.

"He played footsie with me under the table," hissed Binny. "The moment we sat down."

Edward could think of nothing to say. He felt old and tired. He struggled upright and looked down at her, as she rocked backwards and forwards on her haunches in front of the oven. He wondered what he was doing in this dark room, suffering. "I simply can't understand how you managed to lose the pudding," he said. Oh, how he loved her! He confessed it to himself with an anguish that he had never known before. He wanted to put on his coat and leave the house without a word, but he knew he would only succeed in punishing himself. She couldn't run after him and he wouldn't be able to return until tomorrow. She would remain with the Simpsons and list his deceptions and conceits. Far into the night they'd discuss the blemishes of his body and the defects of his mind. They would know he was a silly man.

Excusing himself, he walked down the dark passage to the bathroom and locked the door. He looked at his watch and saw it was five minutes after ten o'clock. Helen would be home at eleven by the latest. He wished he hadn't gone on to that Miriam woman about his garden; describing his wife sitting on a striped deckchair in the sunshine had made him feel uncomfortable, disloyal. There were things he hadn't said. It wasn't only his home-grown vegetables that gave him a sense of achievement; it was having Helen there to appreciate them that counted. Not in a million years would Binny tell him the peas were firm and sweet, and economical into the bargain.

He drew the bolt on the outer door leading to the garden, and flung it wide. The rain bounced on the concrete yard below. Beyond the high wall rimmed with pieces of broken glass, there were cultivated lawns edged with trees; behind the sycamore leaves and the apple blossom, lights shone in the houses. He stepped gingerly on to the little wooden veranda and leaned on the rail. The party wall was crumbling in places. The rambling rose in next door's garden, old and fiercely stemmed, clung to the perished bricks and snaked in an impenetrable thicket along the top. He had tried to encourage Binny to see the possibilities of a town garden. It's no good, she'd said. I can't be bothered. He didn't think he would have done very much himself, for all his talk—a few dwarf roses, a Climbing Caroline, some bulbs in spring. There wasn't the scope for landscape gardening on a grand scale.

He was startled at that moment by a loud knocking on the front door. He gripped the rail of the veranda tightly and stared down at the dark pit of the yard. Who in hell's name could it be? He felt the beat of his heart accelerate wildly. The most dreadful coincidences leapt to his mind. Helen had driven someone home from her meeting, male or female, someone taken frightfully ill —no, not frightfully, they'd have called an ambulance, just unwell. This sick person happened to live in Fulton Street, and damn and blast she hadn't wanted to go home straight away but had decided to visit a friend. That was it . . . this female was often taken ill and this friend of hers had the right sort of medicine. Even now, Helen was on the step supporting this god-awful invalid, and Binny was insisting that both of them should come inside . . .

He looked desperately about the yard, searching for a way of escape. He couldn't climb over the rambling rose; he'd be ripped to pieces. Nor could he manage to straddle the four foot of stout chicken wire that the neighbors on the other side had added to their wall to keep out Binny's children.

He strained his ears listening for voices at the door, footsteps up the hall. His hair was so plastered to his head with rain that drops ran down his cheeks like tears. The house was silent. After a while he relaxed, thinking he must have imagined the sounds. The city was never quiet at night, just as it was never entirely dark. He could see the glow of light that the streets beyond the houses threw up against the sky.

He must break with Binny—the strain was becoming too much for him. He had enough to do as it was, answering phone calls, coping with clients, studying the latest changes in the tax laws. After a tiring day in the office and a visit to Binny in the evening, it was a miracle he didn't drop dead from sheer exhaustion. Sometimes when he returned home, dark rings under the eyes and clothing sprinkled with cat hairs, his wife—allowing her cheek to be brushed by his lips— would suggest that he was doing too much.

Binny had threatened to part with him often enough. Separated from her, he would be like a ship wrenched from its moorings; rudderless, he would be engulfed by enormous waves of grief. He'd have his heart torn out in the process. Binny said No, it wouldn't be like that at all: more like a rowing boat rocking a bit when somebody stood up too quickly. After a couple of seconds the boat would right itself and sit perfectly still: not even a ripple on the water. Of course she was arguing with him at the time—foolishly he'd mentioned some client of his who was having a rough time on twenty thousand a year—and only saying it to hurt him.

For a moment longer he stood staring out at the dripping trees. Then he stepped back inside the bathroom. He rubbed his head vigorously with a towel and, unable to find a comb, raked his hair into place with his fingers. He felt better now, less emotional, restored by the night air. He would take Simpson on one side and suggest they start making excuses about leaving. Perhaps Simpson's back could play him up. He wanted to eavesdrop outside the kitchen door, in case Binny was discussing him, but the house was old and the floor boards creaked at his approach, so he walked straight in.

Alma Waterhouse was lying on the sofa in a deplorable condition.

7

To be fair to Alma, she hadn't wanted to come into the house once she knew Binny had company. She only desired to look at a familiar face and then lie upon the step, quietly weeping.

"Don't be ridiculous," said Binny. "I can't let you stay outside in this state."

"No, no, darling," cried Alma selflessly. "You go back to your party." She leaned against the railings and slid slowly downwards.

Vexed at this dilemma and not sure what to do for the best, Binny was suddenly aware that they were not alone; she peered into the shadows of the hedge. Mrs. Montague was behind the bins again with a friend.

"No, you mustn't," called Binny. "Go away at

once." She seized Alma by the front of her coat and with difficulty pulled her upright. Supporting her round the waist she hauled her up the steps. Mrs. Montague lived further along the street with another friend, who drank a lot; at night he fell unconscious rather than asleep. Mrs. Montague was forced, as she confided to Binny, to take her pleasures where she could, and there wasn't a hedge outside her house. As she was over sixty and far from sprightly, Binny was shocked by her behavior.

"I don't want to be a burden to you," said Alma, once inside the hall. "A smile would have been enough."

"Don't make a noise," whispered Binny. "These people won't like it."

Sniffing, but more composed, Alma entered the kitchen. The warm room, a captive audience, the sight of wine bottles on the table revived her spirits. On being introduced to the Simpsons she smiled indulgently and said, as though pacifying two small children, "Now, darlings. Isn't this nice?"

"She ought to take that coat off," Muriel advised. The woman looked as if she'd been dredged up out of the river.

"I was just passing," Alma said, "And I thought, why not pop in on poor little Binny?" She turned to Simpson. "I've been terribly worried about her, darling."

"Where else have you popped?" asked Binny.

Everything depended on the mood Alma had been in before she started drinking. If she'd felt initially cheerful, and vomiting could be avoided, then she wouldn't prove too difficult to manage.

Alma ignored her. She was wearing her old coat of mock leopard skin and a silk scarf with bedraggled fringes. A false eyelash, partially adrift on her left lid, hung at a raffish angle over one eye; she appeared to be lewdly winking. She spoke again to Simpson, who was appalled by her. He felt that at any moment she was about to say something that might incriminate him. "I've been so worried about her, darling. She's not herself. Wouldn't sit down, wouldn't have a little drinkie . . . must rush off to the shops. And when we got to the shops, she never went near them—"

"I had to go to the bank," said Binny crossly.

"But you didn't stay in the bank, darling. I saw you. You ran in and you ran out. I passed you in a taxi five minutes later and you were down a side street behaving very oddly."

"Take your coat off," snapped Binny. "This minute. And be quiet."

"You could have got run over, darling. Waving your arms about like that." Alma clung to Muriel's elbow to steady herself. "She keeps thinking she's on television, you know."

"I don't do any such thing."

A plaintive, almost childlike expression came over Alma's face. She allowed her lip to tremble. She whispered loudly to Muriel. "She's cross with me. You're not cross, are you? I'm only showing concern."

"I've no reason to be cross," said Muriel, feeling inadequate.

Alma tottered on her feet and squinted reproachfully at Binny. "Why didn't you say your sister was coming? You're so secretive, darling." She and Muriel, joined together at the elbow, took a few little lurching steps across the room.

"You know perfectly well it isn't my sister," said Binny. She stood behind Alma and, jerking the coat from her shoulders, laid it over a chair. Alma was wearing a little red dress with an inch of torn petticoat showing. She spun round with a cry of distress, wounded by the exasperation in her friend's voice and alarmed at the savagery with which her outer garment had been removed.

Muriel put her arms about Alma. Murmuring sympathetically, she began to pat her back. Simpson was astonished. Once at Christmas, his eldest sister Jessie had grown tiddly on vodka and lime. Apart from a fiery complexion and a tendency later to be argumentative at bridge, her inebriation was hardly noticeable. But Muriel had remarked upon the incident for months afterwards, saying how ugly it had been, how positively disgusting; one would have thought poor old Jess had run amok with a samurai sword and spewed up all over the carpet.

For a moment the two women remained in an embrace. When they drew apart there was a slightly malicious smile on Alma's face. She said sorrowfully to Binny, "I've gone through fire and water getting here. I thought you needed me." She collapsed into a chair and laid her cheek against the tablecloth; her hair, darkened by the rain, trailed in the debris of the meal.

"Perhaps a pot of strong coffee would be in order," said Simpson. For some reason he was irritated beyond endurance at the sight of his wife seated beside that boozy female, stroking her bowed head with a tender smile on her lips. And where the devil, he wondered, had Freeman disappeared to?

"I haven't got a sister," Binny told him, going through into the back room to fill the kettle at the sink. "I'm an only child. She knows that perfectly well."

"An only child," repeated Simpson sentimentally, limping from cupboard to draining board in search of cups. "How lonely that sounds."

Alma began to complain about the difficulties she'd encountered coming to Fulton Street. "Those pigs," she said loudly. "Strutting about in their uniforms making their dirty insinuations. If I had my way I'd put them against the wall and shoot the lot of them. I'd shoot the bastards." She raised her head and banged her fist angrily on the table.

"Stop it," cried Binny, running from the stove and removing the vase of carnations out of her reach. "You're knocking food all over the carpet."

"What pigs?" asked Simpson. "Who does she mean?"

"She doesn't like policemen," said Binny. "Her sympathies have always been with the criminal classes."

"Asking me my business," Alma said indignantly. "Demanding to know where I'd been, where I was going. Wanting to take down my address. Crawling along the curb beside me in their nasty little car, trying to intimidate me."

"They're only doing their job," protested Binny. "They probably thought you were a battered wife."

"Oh darling," cried Alma, eyelash askew and cheek dimpled with the imprint of bread crumbs. "How little you know. They're not out to help me. They're far more corrupt than those poor souls robbing jewellers shops and things. I know them. I know them."

"Come now," said Simpson sternly. "We were broken into last year while we were away in the South of France, and the police were marvellous, absolutely first rate." He looked at his wife for affirmation and was outraged to see that she was now holding Alma's hand.

"I pay for their cars you know, darling," said Alma. "Those things with the lights going round on top. We all do. But they don't let me drive a car. They took my licence off me."

"You can hardly blame them for that," Binny said. "In the circumstances."

"Nonsense," cried Alma. "I was perfectly capable. You're not a what's it, you can't possibly judge."

"I bailed her out," explained Binny. She felt more relaxed now that dinner was over. Muriel seemed to be enjoying the drama, and as for Simpson, he was just another Edward—too pompous for words. Men were all alike. It was not being involved with children every hour of the day that made them appear superior. She had only to bear in mind the image of Simpson going into a little cubicle to provide a cloudy specimen and she hadn't the slightest need to feel inferior. "Alma was arguing with her husband and swerving all over the road when this police car came round the corner—"

"I wasn't swerving, darling."

"They booked them and everything, and then Alma said why didn't the policeman take off his clothes, he'd be more comfortable."

Muriel started to laugh.

"He wasn't a policeman, pet. He was a sergeant and very good-looking."

"Drunken driving is a crime," said Simpson stiffly. "It should carry the harshest penalties."

"What are you worried about, darling? I lost my licence, didn't I?" All at once Alma's face crumpled. Tears spilled out of her ludicrous eyes.

"*You* can talk, George," Muriel said coldly. "You're only wearing one shoe."

Alma rose unsteadily from the table and blundered towards the sofa. "I must lie down," she moaned. "I've never been to the South of France." She fell on to the couch. The red dress, too short, rode above her hips. Her black boots, stained by the rain, threshed among the cushions. Keening softly and scrabbling to get into a more comfortable position, she dozed off.

Edward came into the room. Seeing Alma, he hoisted his braces on to his shoulders and asked in a pained voice, "Didn't you tell her we were coming?"

"She had a row with her husband," said Binny. "It wasn't my fault."

"She's too vulnerable," observed Muriel, hovering anxiously about the sofa. "It's in her face. She's like a child dressed up for a party. Underneath is a pure heart struggling to come to terms with life. But then, the way the world is, what chance has she got?"

After this extraordinary question there was silence.

Finally Simpson said, "That's all very fine, but put her behind the wheel of a car and she's lethal. Lethal." He himself thought it was in dubious taste to compare Alma to a child. Granted her eyes and mouth seemed to have been crayoned in by a two-year-old with an unsteady hand, but in every other respect the woman was a tart.

"She's been to the South of France," said Binny. "Several times as a matter of fact. She was a croupier in a casino."

"One more drink," Edward said. "And then we'd better call it a night." He yawned extravagantly. "I've a meeting first thing." His mind was full of facts and figures, sections and clauses, though there was a small space in which he prepared to defend himself, should Binny attack him for leaving too early. He stood at the table and examined the bottles.

"Count me out," said Simpson. What else could he say when he'd been so critical of the sleeping woman, lying there on the couch with the crotch of her knickers showing through her tights? Besides, if he was going to have lunch with his mistress tomorrow he wanted to appear fairly fresh and virile. He didn't approve of the word "mistress" but Freeman had used it first. "I'm just telephoning my mistress," he'd say, or, "I'm seeing my mistress tonight." Once, in the pub, he'd admitted that Binny had slapped his face for using the word. She said only people like Edward VII could invest it with meaning. Unless he was prepared to set her up in a house in the park and send her children to Eton, he should shut up. Actually, thought Simpson, old Freeman appeared to get more of a look in than most. He himself, apart from some heavy petting in his car, had only managed to persuade Marcia to lie down on one occasion. Who the devil was the man who'd answered her phone?

Muriel asked Binny where she had put the fur wrap. "I should like to make her more comfortable," she said, gesturing at Alma, who was now lying on her back with her mouth open.

Simpson raged. He said the coat was too damned expensive to act as a blanket.

The woman looked at him pityingly.

Edward, thinking that fetching the wrap would hasten their departure, directed Muriel upstairs. He didn't offer to accompany her because he didn't want to leave Simpson alone with Binny, and he couldn't go for it himself, seeing there were no curtains at the window and he might be spotted from the street.

In the room above, Muriel was careful not to come into contact with any of the furniture. She was scandalized at the presence of a ping-pong table, whose surface was ringed with the indentures of vanished cups of tea, in a room of such beautiful proportions. It was simply unbelievable. She scrutinized the pictures on the walls. There were various photographs of the same three children from infancy to adolescence. The chubby toddlers smiled, the lean teenagers scowled. There was a wedding portrait of a young Binny in a three-quarter-length dress and a small round hat rimmed with flowers. She was linking arms with a bearded man. Underneath someone had scrawled in pencil "Our Dad, Our Hero." He didn't look like a person who could ever have business commitments. Next to the happy couple hung two framed pictures, cut from magazines, of different men lying in black pools of blood, dying of assassination. There were a lot of books on shelves gray with dust.

Muriel thought it a shame to live in such squalor. No wonder the children didn't appear to be in the house; at a certain age children became very conscious of their surroundings. She could scarcely see out of the unwashed windows—there were pigeon droppings spattered on the glass. Across the road, parked outside the block of flats, waited a police car. It had stopped raining.

She took her fur downstairs and laid it over the hips of Binny's sad friend. Alma was gently snoring.

"There's a car outside," Muriel said. "With two policemen in it. Do you think it's anything to do with her?"

Binny jumped up from the table and went to the window. She began to tug at the bar that kept the shutters in place.

"Don't open them," cried Edward. "Don't encourage them."

"It's hardly likely," Simpson said, "that they'd follow her to the door. I didn't believe a word of that harassment nonsense."

"You don't know Alma," Binny said darkly. "She probably called them every name under the sun. She got deported, you realize, from the South of France."

She sat down again at the table, pleased that she'd alarmed Edward. He was itching to leave—

she'd seen him look twice at his watch in the last five minutes.

They began to talk about France and holidays in general. Edward tried to say as little as possible. Any mention of the two weeks he'd spent with his family in Malta last year would doubtless inflame Binny. It might conjure up visions of his wife lying in the sand, limbs shimmering with *ambre solaire*—of love in the afternoon. In actual fact, most times they'd travelled abroad he'd gone down with a tummy upset on arrival and spent part of each night in the john.

"We've tried Corfu," said Simpson. "It's fairly picturesque. Cricket in the square, pig and chips in the tavernas. Have you tried Corfu?"

"No," Edward said. "Helen's rather tied up, you know—meetings and so forth."

"Meetings?" said Muriel.

"Well, she's on various committees . . . politics . . . schools . . . that sort of thing."

"What schools?" asked Binny. "What sort of thing?"

"She's a school governor," admitted Edward. "And she's secretary of the local Liberal party."

Binny started to have palpitations. She had to put her hand to her mouth to stop abusive words coming out. Though Edward had mentioned on occasions that Helen was at one of her meetings, she had somehow gained the impression that they were to do with the Women's Voluntary Services or even the church. He hadn't hinted that Helen was clever or influential, or in a position of power.

"I've a lot of time for the Liberals," said Simpson.

Binny moved the vase of carnations to one side so that she could see Edward clearly. "Last April," she began, "I was taken out for the day by a gentleman friend. It was terribly exciting for me, as you can imagine. Just for the day, you understand. We went to Yorkshire—"

"It's getting awfully late," Edward said.

"We left London very early in the morning and arrived about eleven. The moment I stepped into the car, I couldn't stand him. I went right off him. I don't know why . . . he just annoyed me—"

"Yorkshire's so pretty," said Muriel.

"I wanted to go to sleep in the car but he wouldn't let me. He kept pointing at trees and boring things like that, as if I'd never seen one before. I was worn out. And then, when we got there, he wouldn't just stop and get out so that we could walk in the country. He kept driving on a little bit further to find somewhere more suitable. It was all suitable to my mind. I couldn't see why, if I wasn't allowed to get out and walk, I couldn't have a bit of shut eye. He was still going on about trees. Anyway, he found somewhere he called suitable and we set off with the sandwiches I'd made. I was terribly hungry . . . I was ravenous—"

"You'd had breakfast," Edward said. "I expect."

"But I wasn't allowed to eat the sandwiches, because that had to be done in a suitable place as well. So I ran off over a field and the next thing I knew this bull started coming towards me—"

"Good God," said Simpson. He was relieved to hear about the bull. He'd feared she was going to divulge all sorts of intimacies in the grass. It couldn't be much fun for old Freeman, listening to tales about her ex-boyfriends. He was looking jolly miserable.

"I ran like hell in the other direction and called this man's name. He wouldn't answer at first . . . he thought I'd come back for the sandwiches. Anyway, to cut a long story short, I felt I'd been a bit rotten and to make amends I asked him about what his uncle did to the grass. He was very fond of this uncle and I thought if I sounded interested he'd be pleased. His uncle used to set fire to tussocks of grass or something. To help the sheep. When it all gets matted and old after the winter, the sheep can't get at the new grass underneath. Have you ever tried to light a fire in the open air?"

"Not often," said Muriel. "As a child perhaps, when camping."

"It's damned difficult," Simpson said. "There's a knack to it. You have to build a kind of tent made out of twigs. It's a question of—"

"Well, I'd never had the knack," continued Binny. "I just idly struck a match and put it to the ground." Dramatically she pursed her lips and made a zipping sound. Her fist shot into the air like a rocket taking off.

The Simpsons stared at her open-mouthed.

"I only did it to be nice to him . . . to show I had faith in his silly old uncle. It was meant as a compliment really. There were sheep having small sheep . . . you know, they were pregnant—"

"Lambing," said Simpson knowledgeably.

"I've never seen anything like it. A little flame ran up the hill like a worm . . . Then the whole field caught fire. There were forests not far away. The police came and six fire trucks from the Forestry Commission."

"How awful," breathed Muriel.

"The sheep went galloping off on those thin little legs, with their stomachs flopping about. This man wouldn't take the blame. I didn't see why we couldn't run for it and drive off in the car. There was too much smoke to read the number plate. He wouldn't . . . He made me own up."

"Was there much damage?" asked Simpson, shocked. He felt enormous sympathy for this unknown man, his bright day ruined by a lunatic woman.

"No," said Binny. "The wind was in the wrong direction. It went out after half an hour." She paused. "He called me a cunt."

Edward cleared his throat. His blue eyes, irritated by his constantly burning pipe, looked sore. He said: "All the men you've known seem to have let you down. One way and another."

Behind him on the sofa, Alma stirred, attempted to sit upright, and was that instant violently sick.

8

Binny and Muriel cleaned up the mess on the carpet. The fur cape, speckled with fragments of undigested food, was shaken out over a piece of newspaper and then dropped inside a large shopping bag.

"I'll take it to the cleaners," Binny promised.

Muriel, thinking in that case she might never see it again, said it didn't matter. The two men, grown pale, were unable to assist.

"I'm so sorry," moaned Alma weakly. "What a nuisance I am. It must have been something I ate." She saw Edward hovering by the door. "Teddy darling," she cried. "Fancy seeing you. Have you had a nice bath, pet?"

Simpson tried to lift up the back window but it was stuck fast. He went into the hall and opened the front door to let out the smell of vomit.

"Look here," whispered Edward, following him. "We really must go home. I'm frightfully late as it is." He shut the door.

"It's not me," said Simpson. "It's my wife. She's well into her Florence Nightingale routine."

Muriel rubbed energetically at the carpet with a piece of rag. When she had finished she rolled the cloth and various soiled tissues into a piece of newspaper and made a parcel of them. Fetching a damp washcloth from the bathroom, she wiped Alma's hands and face. The false eyelash came away.

"My goodness," cried Alma. "It *is* bright in here."

"Muriel," said Simpson, taking her to one side. "Edward wants to leave.'

"Really," she said curtly. "Who's stopping him?"

Alma allowed the stains to be sponged from her red dress. "Is he a friend of yours?" she asked.

"No," said Muriel. "We're married."

Alma began to shiver uncontrollably. The sponging left vivid patches on her breast. Binny wrapped her in one of the children's duffle coats and removed her boots. Eyes filled with remorse and teeth chattering, Alma lay on the sofa with the washing-up bowl placed strategically at her side.

"Oughtn't we to telephone her husband?" asked Muriel.

"Better not," said Binny. "He'll only be obscene."

Muriel picked up the newspaper parcel and took it into the front garden. As she approached the bins she thought she heard voices behind the hedge. Curious, she stepped out on to the pavement. She saw a woman pushing a pram and a taxi coming along the street in the same direction. The woman looked over her shoulder at the taxi, and at that moment the police car on the corner edged into the road. The taxi swerved, scraped the side of Simpson's Fiat parked at the curb and, accelerating, drove left, past the block of flats. The police car reversed, mounted the pavement, rammed a plane tree in a circle of earth and with siren hideously wailing sped round the corner in pursuit. The woman, trundling the pram ahead of her, ran straight at Muriel.

In the front room Edward was standing worriedly at the hearth. What excuse was he going to make to Helen when he arrived home without the Rover? It was getting far too late to collect it from the car park near the office. This wasn't the sort of neighborhood, he knew, much frequented by taxis, and he'd been relying on Simpson, if not to take him back to the City, at least to deposit him at a convenient cab rank. He could hardly come right out with it and ask Simpson to drive him to the car park. He'd always given the impression, he hoped, of being a reckless sort of cove. And Simpson apparently left his own vehicle quite openly in the street when he went to visit his woman in Kilburn. For hours.

How he hated telling too many lies; it brought his face out in blotches. He could have strangled Simpson, dithering there at the sink with a dish towel in his hand and his naked toes exposed. The man was a sissy messing about with dirty plates. He seemed to have forgotten entirely the lateness of the hour. Of course, his wife wasn't sitting at home, waiting to hear his excuses.

Edward looked in the mirror and saw, reflected behind his uncombed head, Jesus on the wall, surrounded by his disciples. It was all right for some, he thought—those who knew the precise moment of their martyrdom. For himself, life stretched ahead, unplanned, full of accidental alarms. The pallor of his face in the glass dismayed him. He recalled the verse of a poem he'd memorized as a boy: "And there lay the rider distorted and pale, With the dew on his brow and the rust on his mail; And the tents were all silent, the banners alone, The lances uplifted, the trumpets unblown . . ."

From somewhere beyond the window he heard the distant clamor of an ambulance. Alma, slumbering within the stifling folds of her khaki duffle coat, whimpered and kicked a cushion to the floor.

Outside the house, still clutching her newspaper package, Muriel stood motionless. The taxi appeared again at the top of the street. The woman stopped running and swivelled the pram sickeningly in a half circle on the wet pavement. The hedge shook. Rain drops slid through the glittering leaves. Dragging the pram behind her, the woman began to mount the steps of Binny's house. The taxi skidded to a halt; men leapt desperately into the road. Muriel moved then and in a dream bent and caught hold of the rubber tires and helped to lift the pram over the top step and into the hall. She was flung bodily toward the stairs. A bicycle rode ahead of her along the carpet and crashed against the bannisters. Hands tore at the hood of the pram; something white, intricate as a paper doily and patterned with light, drifted through the air. She clawed her way back down the hall to where the creeper swayed in the wind. In slow motion, it seemed, she saw an infant, entangled in a crocheted shawl, bounce upon the railings. She screamed. A dimpled knee shone for an instant as a beam of light hurtled across the step. Scooping the limp bundle to her breast, she was seized by the hair and dragged brutally backwards. Falling with arched spine over the hood of the pram, she lost her balance and rolled to the floor; she lay with her cheek pressed to the dark baseboard and the silent baby stuffed within her arms. The front door slammed shut.

To those inside the kitchen, discounting the sleeping woman on the sofa, the sounds from the hall were so sudden and so violent that for several seconds they stood frozen in their tracks. Binny stared at Edward. Her raised hand, arrested between sink and dish rack, gripped a saucer bubbling with soap suds. I love you, she thought. Help me.

Then the door burst inwards.

9

Two men, one dark, one red-headed, held shot-
guns. A third man, unarmed, was gripping a thin
woman by the throat and throttling her.

"The window, Harry," shouted the man with
red hair.

Harry ran to the shutters and punched the
metal bar with his fist. Turning, he swung his gun
in the air like a cricket bat and clouted the yellow
lampshade that hung above the table. The parch-
ment split, the shade pitched wildly; shadows
went bouncing up and down the floor. Edward,
seeing the man's arm rise, ducked instinctively.
For one solitary moment he clung to the illusion
that the pandemonium about him was an elabo-
rate and outragous joke, perpetrated by Binny to

annoy him. Scuttling under the table, he crouched on all fours, watching the man's feet prance upon the carpet.

The third man, having flung his woman victim to the floor, leapt with bent knees on to her chest. She grunted. "Fucking bastard," he screamed.

Chasing the lampshade and jabbing upwards with the sawn-off barrel of his gun, the man called Harry smashed the light bulb. Someone jerked open the shutters. Cautiously Edward crawled backwards towards the wall and stood upright. In the kitchen he saw Simpson and Binny standing motionless, cheek to cheek, as though waiting for a dance orchestra to play.

A tremendous pounding began on the front door. Savagely Edward was gripped by the front of his shirt and thrust against the windows. Bewildered by a curious blue light that flashed across the panes of glass, he stared foolishly into the garden. Black figures milled about the crazy paving. All at once, sighting the pale blur of his face, they swarmed to the railings. Jostling for space on the daffodil border, they shouted words he couldn't understand. Binny and Simpson were hustled to stand beside him. The three of them, aware of guns pointed at their backs, grimaced into the darkness. Binny, trembling with shock, thought only of Edward. Liberated by the fact that her children were not involved, she concentrated entirely on her lover. Knees pressed to the radiator beneath the window ledge, she forgot his failings and his attitudes. The body of Simpson, interposed between them, was an intrusion; her place was at Edward's side. All through dinner she had missed her chance to touch his hand, press his knee. When it came to it, she had given the best chop to Muriel.

She saw Mrs. Montague under the lamplight, holding a bottle of stout in her arms. She was talking to a policeman.

Edward, afraid and alert, visualized Helen in the garden and his son slouching through a gate. He had mistaken familiarity for boredom. Like a landslide, the truths of his childhood, his schooldays, rushed upon him. Play the game, own up, be a man, soldier on. For the second time in his life he had let down the side. God had struck.

In front of the hedge, men held little black boxes to their mouths and communicated with a higher authority.

"What do we do, Ginger?" asked Harry.

By way of answer the red-haired man clubbed the window with the butt of his gun. There was a small stampede as the pane ruptured and pieces of glass spilled into the room.

"Back off," he roared. "Back off."

Outside nobody moved. Mrs. Montague stood with her fist to her cheek. Across the street, crowding the rails of the balconies as though putting out to sea, people waved.

"We've got four of them here," shouted Ginger.

"Bloody well back off." Squeezing Binny by the neck, he ordered, "Tell them your name. Say you live here. Tell them to move, or else."

"My name is Mrs. Mills," cried Binny. "I live here. Please go away." Fearing they might not have heard, she put her mouth to the shattered glass and repeated her request.

Slowly the uniformed men ebbed from the garden and regrouped on the pavement. A whistle blew. Binny's neighbor, the one who was looking after Alison for the night, came to the fence and demanded information. An Alsatian dog on a leather strap leapt round the hedge and nosed the bins.

Ginger closed the shutters.

The room, lit only by a dim bulb hanging above the refrigerator at the kitchen end, seemed touched by moonlight; the edge of a chair shone, a fold of white tablecloth, the bevelled corner of a cardboard invitation stuck in the frame of the mirror. On the wall beneath the electric clock, a red indicator on a power point burned like the butt of a cigarette.

Binny could see Alma sitting bolt upright on the sofa, eyes staring. The men took no notice of her.

"You," said Ginger, looking at Binny. "Is there anyone living upstairs?"

"No one," she said. "Honestly. I promise you."

"Have you got shutters on the first floor windows?"

"Not any more," she said apologetically. "They had woodworm."

"Right," said Ginger. He spoke to Harry. "We don't have to worry about the front door, or the roof. We'd hear the bastards. It's the back and the first floor that needs watching."

The woman lying on the carpet, knees buckled against the lower half of the food cupboard, began to moan. Her assailant stood over her with his hands in his pockets.

"You shouldn't have done that, Widnes," said Harry. He nudged the woman's arm with the toe of his boot.

"Lay off," groaned the woman.

"I want out," the man said. "What in God's name do we do with them?" He indicated the group huddled together in the gloaming of the front room.

"First," Ginger said. "We got to watch the back and upstairs. There's balconies up there. They could climb along from the house next door. Widnes, have a look round the back."

"I want bloody out," repeated Widnes angrily, but already he was going through the door. There was a clatter as he fell over some obstruction in the hall.

The woman sat upright and clutched her ribs. "Crazy bastard," she whined. "He damn near killed me."

"Sod you," said Ginger. He and Harry stood at the back window and peered out at the pink city sky.

"My wife," said Simpson. "Where's my wife?" He went, without interference, to the door. He was ashamed of himself, but he hoped Muriel was still in the house; he didn't want to be left alone.

Muriel was sitting on the stairs holding a doll on her knee. She was playing with its celluloid toes and frowning.

"Where have you been?" asked Simpson. He became terribly angry at the thought of her hiding in the hall when he had been exposed to such violence. The skirt of her dress, he noticed, was streaked with dirt and torn at the hem.

"I was out at the bins," she said. "Seeing to Alma."

"I told you not to bother with that woman," he scolded. "You made a ridiculous fuss of her."

"I was glad of something to do," Muriel said. "I'm used to doing things for you and the children. It's what I'm for. I don't know what to do with my hands when I'm not busy. After the children were walking and we gave the pram away, I used to cross my arms over my chest when I went out."

"Look at the state of your dress," shouted Simpson. "And your stockings. You realize your fur is ruined. It's in the most disgusting mess, absolutely disgusting."

"Stop it," she said. "I'm frightened."

He sat on the stairs beside her and put his arms round her shoulders. There were smashed picture frames on the carpet and pieces of broken glass. Where the bicycle had leaned there was now a dark blue pram; the handlebars of the bicycle were twisted and caught in the bannisters.

"I've seen one of them before," said Simpson. "The one called Widnes."

"Why are they here?" Muriel asked. She looked down at the doll and let it fall on the stair. "I thought it was real," she said.

"They won't harm us," said Simpson. "There's too many of us. What would be the point? Whatever they've done, it couldn't be worth shooting the lot of us." He thought of the woman on the floor, battered by the man he'd met at the telephone kiosk. It was a mercy he hadn't argued with the fellow over who should first use the phone.

Ginger came into the hall. "Inside," he shouted, pointing his gun at Simpson's knees. He dragged the pram backwards into the kitchen and felt underneath the storm cover. Taking out a revolver, he gave it to Harry. The two of them left the room.

The woman was now sitting on a chair by the sink, holding a shotgun on her lap. The pram stood beside her. Gripping the handle in one hand and staring sullenly ahead, she began idly to push it back and forth.

10

Alma was the first to speak. She whispered into the half darkness. "What's it all mean, darlings? I thought you were playing silly games. All that banging about. Why don't you sit down?"

Nobody answered her.

She crawled along the sofa and poked her head round the cupboard. "You don't mind if they sit down, do you, dear? They've had a shock."

"Sit at the table," ordered the woman. "But don't go near the sodding door."

Binny sat on Edward's knee and clung tightly to his neck. He felt comforted by her warm body on his lap and her breath fanning his cheek. In the circumstances it didn't matter any more about keeping up appearances for Muriel's sake. He tried to think when and how Helen would know where he was. There wasn't a phone number in his diary, or any little pieces of incriminating paper in the pockets of his other suits. She'd look up Simpson's number in the directory, he supposed, but that wouldn't help. He didn't imagine Simpson would have told his daughters where he was going; they were both over eighteen and possibly out themselves. Helen would ring the hospitals first and later the police. It would take hours to get through to the casualty wards—it was practically impossible to find anyone on duty even in an emergency. By the time she'd finished her inquiries, they might be released and free to go home. He'd have to make a statement of course, but these days the police were very understanding. He could even say he'd been passing the house and decided to give chase. The police were always inciting the public to have a go. Or maybe he was on the premises at Simpson's invitation. He could mention he'd been taken ill—something like a heart attack. He'd lie merely to Helen, not to the police—that would be irresponsible and wrong. God knows, he wouldn't have to fake it— he felt like death.

"Can I sit with them, dear?" said Alma. "I feel a bit out of it over here."

The woman didn't reply. Keeping a wary eye on the shotgun, Alma moved from the sofa to sit at the table. She was still wearing the duffle coat with its hood pulled over her head. She looked like an under-sized monk, the tip of her nose showing and her hands lost in a welter of sleeves.

Overhead footsteps sounded on the wooden floor. Furniture was being dragged across the room.

"I don't suppose this will go on for very long," said Edward. "They've got procedures worked out for this sort of situation. There's been so much of it lately."

Alma was anxious to know what sort of situation it was. Having been asleep at the time, somewhat under the weather as she freely admitted, she wasn't absolutely sure what had occurred. Like a bird, eyes bright, beaked nose dipping above the tablecloth, she peeped from the hood of the duffle coat.

"Hostages," explained Edward. "It's obvious. They've escaped from somewhere. Some jail. It happens all the time."

"But how can they be hostages, darling?"

"Lower your voice," snapped Simpson. "Not them. Us."

Alma looked at him. "You were horrid to me before," she said. "Yes you were, pet, don't deny it." She waggled her sleeve at him flirtatiously.

Edward spoke in low undertones of a decaying society, the gradual breaking down of law and order, overcrowded prisons, lack of money. There was no doubt about it, they were living in decadent times. He was conscious that no one followed his train of thought. "Why, only last week," he confessed, "I was undercharged at the chemists. Helen had a twinge of neuralgia and I went to buy aspirins. I don't hold with aspirins myself. Do you know, I pocketed the surplus change without a word. I'm not proud of my action, but I did."

"Why couldn't she buy her own aspirins?" asked Binny. She would have liked to move from Edward's knee, but there was nowhere else to sit.

"They can't have been in much of a hurry to get away," said Simpson. "I've seen one of them before. Hours ago when I went to fetch the wine from the car."

They sat hunched over the table, talking softly, pushing knives and forks across the cloth and playing with small crumbs of bread. Those initial minutes of violence receding into the past, they were like travellers previously lost in a blizzard who found themselves safe for the moment beside the fire. Muriel alone crouched silent in her chair; now and then her eyes strayed to the blue pram in the kitchen. Alma was incensed, on Binny's behalf, at the broken window and the mutilated lampshade. In her view such vandalism was quite unnecessary. She had run away from her own home earlier in the evening because her husband, unable to find any clean socks for the morning, had called her a slut and thrown the milk jug at her. She was willing to admit she'd been remiss— though they weren't her socks and he hadn't as far as she knew an allergy to soap—but he'd given her no time before taking aim.

"I've a good mind to have a word with that Harry man," she said. "It was very naughty of him. Men never think of the mess they make."

"Good Lord, don't," warned Edward, full of misgivings. "It's quite the wrong attitude to take. We have to strike up a rapport . . . It's a question of psychology . . . We're all in it together. At the same time we must strive to achieve a certain delicate balance between abject cooperation and some degree of firmness. There must be no aggravation, but on the other hand we shouldn't crawl . . . if you follow me. We should endeavor to show them what's what—"

Alma smiled.

"I've read about it," he said defensively. "It's vital not to seem hostile."

"Don't be silly, Ted darling. They're no different from you and me. They've just got caught up in an everyday problem that's gone a teeny bit wrong."

Edward began to bluster. He found Alma infuriating, quite apart from the way she addressed him. He jiggled Binny up and down on his agitated knees. "It may be an everyday problem to you, but personally I'm not used to being hijacked in my own home by armed thugs."

"Here, here," said Simpson.

"They're alien to us," insisted Edward. "It's a

different breed, a different culture."

Binny put her lips to his temple. His hair smelt of tobacco. She knew he had made a slip, thinking this was home, but all the same it was nice of him. At the back of her mind she thought she was making a fuss of him for somebody else's benefit. To gain attention.

Edward jerked his head away; he was trembling. Surely it was perfectly natural to go for aspirins if one's wife was feeling groggy. One would do it for the dog. None of them knew each other well enough, that was the difficulty. They were all behaving in an unreal manner. He couldn't count on their reactions under stress. One of them was potentially dangerous—it might even be himself.

Simpson said, "Mussolini used to say, whenever I hear the word culture I reach for my gun."

"Exactly," cried Alma, though she didn't know what he meant.

"Be quiet," said Muriel. She was staring into the kitchen.

They stopped breathing and looked fearfully at the woman by the sink. She had ceased to roll the pram and was now hunched over the shotgun, nursing her ribs.

Binny felt she was taking part in some sort of documentary—one of those programs that used members of the public and portrayed ordinary lives from a melancholy point of view. She realized she'd been in it right from the moment she went shopping with Alma. Those old ladies posed on the bed down the alleyway . . . the waitress in the Wimpy Bar so reluctant to serve them. The woman in the chair was the character who'd left her pram outside the bank. She wasn't instantly recognizable because her face was altered by that scene in which she'd been battered; her stockings were a different color. They'd been shooting her from various camera angles in the National Westminster, that's why she kept moving from queue to queue at the counter. The black man with his neck in plaster also fitted in somewhere.

"Why has she changed sides?" Simpson whispered. He thought the woman must be incredibly fit. Had he been treated half as brutally he was sure he would have succumbed from shock. He recalled his mother who had taken to her bed every afternoon, prostrate from a fatiguing morning spent attending to the furniture with a feather duster. His aunts had been the same—fragile, languid. He thought of Marcia living with two men, and Muriel quite capable of pushing the car singlehanded round the block, when it was a cold morning and the engine wouldn't start. It was a generation of Amazons.

"She hasn't changed sides," hissed Binny. "She's the same side but she's double-crossed them or something. She was on the wrong route. She tried to explain it to them but they wouldn't listen. They were looking for her."

"They don't have mixed prisons," Alma said.

"She must be an outside contact. She probably had a change of clothing for them in the pram."

Edward had come to the conclusion that the guns couldn't be loaded; they were purely for intimidation purposes. That particular type of weapon, with the barrel sawn off, was surely more suited to gang warfare than for going over the wall.

"He's awfully sweet," Alma said into Binny's ear. "You shouldn't be so cross with him, darling. It's quite natural to go to the chemist."

Ginger and Harry entered the room. Edward caught himself nodding. It was like growing familiar with people on the television—actors, celebrities—and then seeing them on the tube or in a restaurant. One imagined one knew them socially.

Harry was holding his hands distastefully in front of him. "It's bloody disgusting up there, missus," he said. "Don't you believe in cleaning?" He went to the sink and turned the tap full on.

Despite his rudeness Binny wondered if she should offer to make a cup of tea. It wouldn't be a fawning gesture—more of a cooperative one, in line with Edward's suggestion.

Ginger murmured something into the woman's ear. She put the gun down on the draining board and attempted to pull herself upright.

"You're breaking my heart," cried Ginger. "Stop playing silly buggers."

Kicking off her high-helled shoes and wincing

with pain, the woman succeeded in standing.

"What about them?" asked Harry.

"Christ," Ginger said. "They're all past it. We've landed in an old people's club." He looked scornfully at the group around the table. "Stay exactly where you are," he told them, "and you won't get hurt." He followed Harry and the woman into the hall and shut the door.

"Of course, it's dark," observed Alma, after a moment's silence. "And I've got this dreadful coat on." She struggled with the toggles at the front. "What on earth possessed you to wrap me in this thing, darling?"

"You'd been sick over everything else," Binny said. She was trying to hold in her stomach muscles. She had never pretended to be younger than she was. There was hardly any gray in her hair and sometimes in the warm weather, in a summery outfit, people remarked how juvenile she looked. She glanced at Muriel. She was somewhat thick about the waist and her make-up was elderly —powdered cheeks and pencilled brows—but she wasn't decrepit by any means. Ginger was probably referring to Simpson and Edward, with their beer bellies and their old men's suits.

"I'm frantic to spend a penny," said Edward. He squirmed in his seat and the rickety chair swayed under him. He remembered a newspaper report he'd read about people being locked up in a vault for several days. The article hadn't spelled it out in so many words, but reading between the lines it was obvious everyone peed into a communal bucket. Some men, he realized, rather went for that sort of carry on—women squatting, tinkling into chamber pots and so forth. He himself grew faint with nausea at the prospect.

"We ought," said Simpson, looking directly at Edward, "to be thinking of a way out of this mess. Just in case your cooperation theory doesn't work. I'd like to have an alternative plan up my sleeve."

"I never suggested total cooperation—"

"It's true," said Binny loyally. "He did mention firmness as well."

"I don't altogether care for being firm," said Simpson. "Not when I'm under armed guard. What I propose is that we try to create some kind of diversion and then one of us should make a break for it."

Edward stared at him appalled. "I don't really see what good that would do. It would have to be me or you and that would leave the women with very little protection."

"Any minute," said Simpson, stabbing the tablecloth with his finger, "they could start separating us. Taking away our sense of unity. You upstairs, Binny in the bathroom, the rest of us scattered elsewhere, bound and gagged."

"Do stop it," protested Edward. "Can't you see you're alarming the girls?"

"What sort of diversion?" asked Alma with interest. She was thinking of a film she'd seen in which prisoners of war gave a concert party while under the stage a tunnel was being dug.

"There's a back door," Binny said helpfully. "It leads into the garden."

"It's quite impossible," cried Edward. "There's broken glass on one wall and a wicked rose on the other. You wouldn't stand a chance."

"He might have meant you," said Binny. "You could go." She didn't really mean it and would much rather have Simpson take any risk that was called for, but it was like those rare occasions when she visited relatives with the children and they refused to help with the washing-up or to talk about O levels. One was forced to show them up.

"Out there," said Edward, "the police are watching our every move." He pointed dramatically at the shuttered windows. "They know everything that's going on. They have manpower, resources, know-how. The most sophisticated areas of psychology and technology are being explored and utilized. They don't need us to throw a spanner in the works. They can probably hear every word we say."

The women looked at him, impressed. Aware that he had their full attention, he struggled upright. Dumping Binny on her feet, he strode to the fireplace and tapped the wall authoritatively; he felt like a military instructor pin-pointing the danger spots on the globe. "Behind there they are taping our conversations. Every sentence we utter. We don't need to endanger our lives to pass on information, we have merely to speak to the wall."

"I don't believe it," said Simpson skeptically. "They'd need to push wires through the bricks. We'd have heard noises." He wished to God Freeman would stop playing head boy. It was bloody irritating under the circumstances.

"The sort of device I'm thinking of is far more advanced than that," Edward informed him severely. "You'll have to take my word for it. We really mustn't have any more foolish talk about diversions, and mock heroics in the backyard." It was imperative, he thought, to nip Simpson's ridiculous bid for escape in the bud. The man was itching for glory and only thinking of himself. While he was gallivanting over walls, others would be left to cope with his wife.

Alma tiptoed to the hearth. She leaned against the flowered wallpaper and whispered urgently to a leaf, "Hallo, hallo. Are you there? Over and out." She waited. "Is it similar to that thing at the doctor's?" she asked Edward. "When he listens to your chest?"

"Same principle," he agreed. He returned to the table and like a conscientious mother scooped Binny once more on to his knee. "I feel so damned uncomfortable," he confided miserably, nuzzling into the dark curls on her neck. Deep down he was thinking that no technological breakthrough on earth was going to remove the pressure on his bladder, or make Helen understand what he was doing in a house she'd never heard of when he'd implied he was going to Simpson's office. Part of him, now that midnight had passed, welcomed an extended imprisonment. The longer he remained captive the better; it would give Helen time to come full circle from anger to relief. With any luck she'd be so grateful finally at his release, that she wouldn't insist on divorce. I've been a fool, he heard himself telling her. But by God I've paid for it.

"You wouldn't need to make holes in the brick," said Alma, kneeling on all fours and putting her head in the grate. "They could dangle a little bug thing down the chimney." She felt about in the darkness for wires.

Simpson averted his eyes from her buttocks. He said stubbornly, "I'm not prepared to sit here and do nothing. Personally it won't give me any satisfaction at all to know my groans are being recorded when I'm trussed up like a turkey. I want to know the lay-out down there."

"Down where?" asked Binny.

"The garden. How many steps are there into the garden?"

"Six," said Binny, after some thought.

"Eight," corrected Edward. He detested inaccuracy.

"And what's at the bottom of the steps? Flower pots . . . garden furniture?"

"There's nothing," Binny said. "Except for a

rabbit hutch against the back wall. It's just a yard."

Alma returned to the table and told them that when she was little she thought Father Christmas lived up the chimney. "My Uncle Len used to stand in front of the fire on Christmas eve and shout in a funny voice, 'Are you all right, Father Christmas? Not too hot, I hope?' Isn't it silly, darlings, what you think of?"

"I can't remember its name," mused Edward. "Tiger . . . Twinkle . . . something like that."

If they really were listening to every word, thought Simpson, the police would think they were cracking up. When he got out of this, even if it was dawn, he was going to go straight round to Marcia's and find out who had answered the telephone. The lunches he'd bought her, the bottle of perfume he'd sent on her birthday, the time he'd wasted when he should have been attending to his business! He wondered sadly if she found bald men unattractive. Muriel had once told him he was better-looking now than when she'd first met him. But then, when she'd met him, Marcia hadn't been born. How the devil had she known he was in a call box?

"The gun," Muriel said. "On the draining board."

They stared bewildered at the weapon not six feet away. "It proves my point," Edward said uneasily. "They wouldn't leave a loaded gun lying around."

"They're under a considerable strain," reminded Simpson. "Particularly that poor girl." He was acutely aware of his wife, sitting there in the shadows in an attitude of childlike passivity, detached from the general discussion yet capable of noticing such things. She was behaving oddly. Usually in a crisis—the girls late home, a minor accident to the car—she was prone to bossiness, to taking control. He'd tried twice in the last half hour to comfort her; each time she'd removed her cold hand from beneath his and withdrawn it to her lap. He sensed she was watching, waiting, and it unnerved him. "I think you ought to have a go at it, Freeman," he said. "Your background and all that."

"Look here, I never saw any action, you know."

"I meant the ducks, old man. That sort of thing."

"They told us we mustn't move," whispered Binny. "They said we'd better not." All the same she loosened her arms from about Edward's neck.

"I'll provide a cover," offered Simpson, as Edward rose reluctantly from his chair. He began to mutter absurdly, "Rhubarb, rhubarb, rhubarb..."

The floorboards creaked as Edward tiptoed laboriously towards the kitchen. Though he was inching his way with obsessive caution, one foot placed carefully in front of the other, it was as if he was running full tilt across the room. It was similar to those agonizing moments in the school gymnasium, when it was his turn to vault the horse. Any second now he was doomed to spring upwards and attempt the splits in mid-air. Perspiration began to trickle down the collar of his shirt. He should never have mentioned those beastly birds. He peered at the gun from several angles, bottom thrust to the group in the other room, heart thumping lest Harry should return—or worse, the inhuman brute who had leapt upon the woman. To his relief the gun was lying on a bed of upturned plates. Moving considerably faster on his return journey to the table, he explained that the whole thing was rather like a house of cards. The weapon was lodged among dishes and things. One false move and the whole caboodle would fall with a fearful clatter into the sink. If the women hadn't been present he might have been prepared to take the risk. As things stood he simply couldn't take the responsibility for a confrontation at this point. They could all be shot down like flies. "You see my dilemma," he said, hovering thankfully about the table.

"But you said the guns wouldn't be loaded, pet."

"We can't be certain. Not one hundred per cent certain."

Binny made no move to let him sit again. He was forced to lean against the wall, fists clenched to the pit of his stomach.

"Loaded or not," Muriel remarked. "It won't make any difference. They don't mean us to live."

11

Outside, the police were requesting householders to remove their cars from the street. Several women in torn nightclothes dragged deck chairs onto the balconies.

A confused report had come in regarding a woman and two children held for six hours in a house in Wood Green and just released. Nothing had been verified, but someone higher up thought that the events in Wood Green and the uprising in Fulton Street might be connected. A baby's shawl had been found on the railings and the tracks of pram wheels on the pavement.

The taxi, abandoned with open doors in the middle of the road, was briefly scrutinized and then photographed. Later a breakdown van arrived to take it away for more serious examination. There was a subdued round of applause from spectators as the taxi was hoisted into the air, doors swinging, and lowered gently on to the bed of the truck. Inquiries were made and statements taken. A dishevelled Mrs. Montague, spitting with excitement, told of a crying female sprawled on the step earlier in the evening, of a lady in a blue frock holding a suspicious-looking parcel in her arms. A youth across the road swore he'd seen a man with a wooden leg dragging himself toward the garage at about nine o'clock. Several people recalled a shortish individual in a suede overcoat, prowling up and down the steps of houses and behaving like a Peeping Tom.

The neighbors on either side of Binny were warned they might have to be evacuated. It was not clear what was going on inside the barricaded house, or how many persons were involved, but investigations were under way. Sybil Evans answered the questions put to her as discreetly as she was able. She was shy and hated explicit conversation. She had known Mrs. Mills for a number of years—they were friendly, not close. It was a popping-in-and-out sort of relationship—borrowing things, feeding cats when one or other of them went away on holiday. Loyally she forbore to mention that it was Binny who did the borrowing. Two older children were staying with friends and the youngest child was upstairs sharing the back bedroom with her own daughter.

When asked if she thought any significance could be attached to the absence of all the children from the house, she was nonplussed. "Well," she said weakly. "there's a dinner party, I believe, and she wanted the house to herself." As she spoke, she realized she'd implied that Binny might have been planning some kind of orgy. "They're large children," she added. "Noisy and hard to control." She hadn't been told who was coming to dinner and she hadn't asked. It was none of her business. She had no objection to a policewoman asking the youngest child for information, but not until the morning—the little girl was fast asleep and it was going to be difficult enough to cope with her when she woke; she was very attached to her mother. To her knowledge Binny wasn't in the habit of entertaining formally—people dropped in for a drink, but she didn't hold dinner parties. She had no idea why tonight had been an exception. There was a gentleman friend, but she hadn't met him and she didn't know his name. "Please," she said finally, "I don't wish to say any more." Pressed, she admitted she'd glimpsed Binny that morning throwing something down into the yard. Only for a second. Her interrogators wanted to know how Binny had seemed. Was there anything unusual about her, peculiar—? With some spirit she declared that anyone would appear peculiar in these particular circumstances. "Life itself is peculiar," she cried. Willingly she described the interior of Binny's house, the position of the furniture. She allowed an assortment of men, uniformed and otherwise, to bring their equipment into the hall. Painstakingly they began to measure the dimensions of the rooms.

12

There was talk of tying Edward and Simpson to their chairs with rope. Simpson glanced accusingly at Edward but said nothing. The gunmen were worried that with Widnes in the bathroom and Ginger upstairs, it left only Harry to deal with a possible rebellion in the kitchen. Their injured confederate was unlikely to move fast in an emergency. Binny said she didn't own any rope.

"You needn't worry about us, dears," Alma told them. "We shan't be any trouble."

"Don't you have a washing line?" asked Ginger. "Where do you hang your stuff?"

"I go to the bagwash down the road," Binny admitted. "There's a spin-drier. I don't need to put it in the yard." Years ago she had pegged the clothes out to dry in the back, but it was such a business tripping down the steps that she kept forgetting where she'd put the jeans and the pajamas. When she did remember, they were either wetter than ever or stiff with frost. In the summer the soot from the factory chimney two streets away drifted like pollen across the gardens. She'd stopped bothering.

Harry went upstairs and brought down a sheet from the divan bed. Binny thought he was going to say it was a disgraceful color, but he made no comment. He tore it into strips and sat Edward under the bulb in the kitchen. Binny felt possibly the government would give her money to buy new linen—there must be some kind of compensation for a situation like this, unless it came under an act of God.

Edward's legs were tied together at the ankles. He found himself smirking with embarrassment as he helpfully stretched his feet in front of him. There was a moment, he realized, when everything was too late, but he couldn't be sure which moment it was. It may already have passed. It would be foolish to be beaten insensible for nothing. They tied his wrists behind his back and finally he was tethered to the chair itself with several bands of sheeting.

"Move about," said Ginger.

Edward did as he was told.

"More," Ginger commanded.

Red in the face, Edward lunged obediently backwards and forwards. The chair fell apart. As he jerked his arms involuntarily to save himself from hitting the floor, the cotton bandages gave way.

"Christ Almighty," cried Ginger. His grip tightened on his gun.

Edward wet himself.

13

Binny woke thinking she heard children crying. She remained for several seconds with eyes shut, cheek pressed to the rumpled tablecloth. She identified the sound as that of cats yowling somewhere beyond the back yard. Still, her heart continued to beat fast with terror. She thought of a little girl, in the dark and afraid, standing in ankle socks on brown linoleum, wailing for her Mummy. Tears came to her eyes. When the children were younger and one of them had a feverish temperature, she was reduced to the same state of mind as if the child were already dead. If they were late home from school, dallying at the ice cream van, she imagined them lying in the center of the road, vanilla cones upended in the dust, stricken down by some heavy vehicle. Sometimes she would torture herself with images of small coffins heaped with flowers and find herself at tea-time standing at the window, staring mesmerized at the bright blue sky, humming fragments of hymns learned long ago on Sunday afternoons. When in the first years of her marriage she had confided these unhappy thoughts to her husband, he hadn't understood. It was like wading through mud to reach him. "Don't be silly, love," he'd said. "Don't be morbid." Finally, worn down by such graphic descriptions of her maternal feelings, he had laughed uneasily and called her a neurotic bitch. She was sure he was right.

Raising her head, she looked emotionally about the room. Alma and Muriel lay upon the sofa, wheezing as they slept. As if hurled from a fast-moving train, they sprawled in grotesque disorder, pale legs entwined, sunk within the hollow of the couch. There was no sign of Edward or Simpson.

Earlier, Ginger had lined them up along the hall and allowed them to go singly into the bathroom. He'd kept the door ajar. Edward, for whom it was too late, had remained in the kitchen. When herded again into the front room, Binny had wanted to lie down on the floor with him and rest, but he'd refused. "I stink," he'd said forlornly. "Leave me alone."

"I don't care," she'd cried. "You're fragrant as apple blossom to me."

"For God's sake," he'd said, and turning away had sat down beneath the shuttered windows with his back to the radiator and closed his eyes.

After a time Simpson had joined him. They slumped shoulder to shoulder, heads lolling, and drifted into sleep. Edward's pipe had fallen to his lap. Binny had placed it carefully on the table. She would have liked to hold it to her heart, but its smell affected her.

The pipe had gone. She knelt and searched for it on the floor. When she stood up the tips of her fingers were stained with pink. She persuaded herself that it was wine not blood, standing there with her hand extended toward the light of the kitchen as though she were Lady Macbeth. Trembling, she went into the hall. Propped against the front door sat the injured woman, chin on her breast and gun laid across her knee.

Binny climbed the stairs and went into the bedroom. She stopped motionless on the threshold of the door, bewildered by the moon. She had been so long entombed in the dimly lit kitchen that she was unprepared for the sweetness of the air she breathed, the stretch of stormy sky beyond the windows, milky with light, filled with white clouds ballooning high above the roof tops. She felt that the room too was drifting in space, dappled with the shadows of leaves, of railings, and turning, turning . . .

"What's up?" said Ginger, "What's Harry want?"

"Nothing," she said. "He's asleep by the stove. What have you done to the gentlemen? What's happened to Edward?"

"Is he the one that pissed hisself?" he asked. The large table had been dragged across the room and laid on its side to form a barricade. Ginger crouched behind it. The tip of his gun glittered like a spear in the moonlight.

"He wasn't scared," defended Binny. "He couldn't hold on any longer. Where is he?"

"In the bathroom. They're all right."

"Someone's bleeding," she accused. "There's blood on the carpet."

"The bald bloke hurt his ankle," Ginger said. "It had nothing to do with us."

Binny advanced further into the room. She noticed a pane of glass had been broken in the bottom half of the window. She looked curiously into the street. It was empty of cars, of people; lights burned on the stairwells of the flats and along the deserted balconies. At the corner, by a plane tree turned to silver under the blazing moon, a solitary furniture van was parked. "What would you have done," she wanted to know, "if the children had been here? My children?"

He shrugged.

"They'd have been frightened."

"They'd have been asleep," he said sullenly. "Wouldn't they?"

"Alison watches late-night films sometimes. She could have been up."

He said nothing. He was like her son Gregory when she started to tell him how tired she felt; his mind switched off.

"You shouldn't involve other people. It's none of my business what you've been doing, but you shouldn't have brought it here. You don't know how inconvenient it is."

"Shut up," he said. "I never asked to be here."

"Alison would have been frightened out of her wits. Smashing the pictures in the hall, fusing the lights—"

"We never fused them."

"Beating that woman—"

"You know nothing about it," he muttered. "It's not what you think."

"Children are very impressionable. It's like food—we are what we eat. They can be influenced for life. It doesn't matter to us . . . we've had our lives."

He stared at her. She couldn't see his expression.

"Well," she amended. "You haven't, of course. You're only young. You won't remember that film, will you, when the heroine walked into the ocean playing her violin? She said more or less the same thing. That's why she did it."

She didn't worry whether Ginger thought the strain of the last few hours had unhinged her; she was choosing her words with care. Far away, like a distant gust of wind, she heard those fornicating cats, thinly screaming. She was ready at the slightest hint of irritation on his part to change her attitude, to moderate her tone of voice. She would never have spoken in this fanciful way to Harry or the violent man in the bathroom. They were not the same as Ginger. For many years, in the privacy of her own home, she had been a voyeur of murder, arson and war. Sitting passively on her sofa she had followed in the wake of tanks and ships and planes. She had seen shells burst in the night like fireworks, flame-throwers curling like rainbows above the earth. She had watched little bombs falling, wobbling like harmless darts through fluffy clouds. Between placing the kettle on the gas and the water coming to the boil, whole cities disintegrated, populations burned. A thousand deaths, real and fictional, had been enacted before her eyes. Once, in real life, she'd been an innocent bystander when a woman was attacked with an axe. Head elongated, wearing a bloody rag of a towel like an Indian turban, the victim was helped from the house. Binny found the moans simulated, the suffering unconvincing; the scene lacked reality, the woman lacked star quality. Ginger's voice, and that bowed head theatrically lit by moonlight, were familiar to her. She could believe in him. He was the wayward young man in westerns and gangster movies and war films who at the end, sickened by his less stylish companions, proved to have a heart of gold.

"I don't want to know the details," she continued. "What you've done, you've done. That's your affair. But you ought to tell us what you're going to do next. After all we're on your side whether we like it or not. Why on earth did you have to break this window?" She bent down fussily and inspected the fragments of glass on the dusty floor.

"I kept dozing off," he explained. "It wouldn't open. I needed air."

"Yes, well," she said. "That's one way of getting it, I suppose. The paint's stuck. There's so much to do in a house this size. I can't be expected to do everything." She gazed, consumed with self-pity, into the street below. "They've left us alone," she lamented. "Not one single bobby. They don't care what happens to us."

"Don't you believe it," Ginger said. He pointed at the van on the corner. "That's their H.Q. And there's men up there."

"Where?" she asked. She squatted beside him and peered intently over the edge of the table. "Those are birds, surely?"

"There," he said impatiently. He held her chin and tilted it in the right direction.

His fingers were thin and strong; she could feel his breath upon her cheek. She wasn't worried by his proximity. It wasn't only that he regarded her as eligible for the old age pension; she'd enough knowledge of men to know he couldn't fancy her. "Oh yes," she cried, "I see," though all she saw on the slopes of the moon-flooded roof were pigeons perched in sleep.

"I keep thinking of steak," said Ginger. "I thought I heard it spitting under the grill a moment ago."

"We haven't got any steak," she said.

"It's those leaves on the balcony," he told her. "That ivy, flickering against the railings."

"There's some sausages in the fridge. You're very welcome."

He made a face. "Muck," he said contemptuously.

She hoped he was referring to sausages in general. After Harry's disparaging remarks about cleanliness she was unduly sensitive. She looked at him. There were creases at the side of his mouth. He wasn't as young as she'd first taken him to be—perhaps prison life had aged him. "Was it awful inside?" she asked.

They stayed like two monkeys on the floor, balanced on haunches, hands swinging loosely between their knees.

He stared at her blankly. "Inside where?"

"Well, prison."

"How should I know?" he said. "I never been there."

"No, of course not," she agreed. "I was just curious." He had a surprised kind of face, the eyebrows so pale as to be unnoticeable. His lips couldn't quite close over his teeth. He looked good-tempered and expectant, as though waiting for some joke to be told. "I've visited me brother, though. In Walton."

"Is that a prison?"

"Yes," he said. "It's a good few years ago now."

"It must be terrible to be shut away. It must finish a man."

"Get off," he scoffed. "You don't know what you're talking about. Our Billy never looked fitter in his life. When I went to see him you'd have mistaken the blokes inside for the visitors. It was me and me sister looked half-dead."

"That's interesting," said Binny.

"Stands to reason, doesn't it? They put him to bed at eight o'clock and he had a bath three times a week. He got into music and foreign languages. He sat up half the night with his earphones."

"How amazing," said Binny.

"You ask our Billy anything about Mahler and Stravinsky and he'll tell you. Anything at all. He knows them backwards."

She was resentful. She recalled the times she'd tried to listen to Vera Lynn on the gramophone and Sybil Evans' curtailing her with a knock on the bedroom wall.

"It's another world," she said. "I can't pretend to understand." She couldn't think what else to say. She didn't like to ask him what he was doing in her house if he hadn't escaped from prison. It wouldn't do to irritate him, not when they were getting on so well. "Look," she said. "Why don't

I go downstairs and make us all something to eat? There's brown bread and some nice cheese. That would do you good. It's wholemeal bread. Then you could tell us what's happening . . . you know . . . put us in the picture. Edward's awfully upset." She hesitated, wondering how much to tell him.

"Your hubby?" Ginger said. "The fat bloke?"

"He's not that fat," she protested. "It's only his stomach. He eats a lot and sits down all day." Ginger was watching the street, the roof opposite, the furniture van on the corner. "You see he's not really supposed to be here. He's a kind man, a good man. He is, really. I know he sounds pompous and he's a bit crippled by being educated at that posh school, but he'd never let anybody down. He's got values. I haven't got values." She could feel her lip beginning to quiver. "That's why the children take no notice of me. I don't give them a lead. Alison takes notice of me —she gives me cuddles, but then she's only a baby. Edward's different from me. He's got a wonderful sense of responsibility. It weighs him down. And he's awfully brave. Why, when he went for the gun—"

"What gun?" asked Ginger.

"When he was little," she improvised. "He had this nanny who kept pushing her babies in the mud. Though he was only a boy he got his gun out and stopped her. It was very brave."

"What mud?" Ginger asked.

"In the country. It rained all the time. Of course, it was his background. He has this thing about playing the game and keeping a stiff upper lip."

"He didn't have a stiff upper anything a couple of hours ago," Ginger said cruelly.

"Don't," she pleaded. "You shouldn't make fun of him. I can't see why you don't let him go. He's like a fish out of water. You could just shove him through the front door. He won't give away any information, not if he gives you his word. He's like that."

"No," Ginger said.

"What difference would it make?"

"I'll say this for you," remarked Ginger. "You're loyal. You stand by your bloke."

"He's married," she confessed. "He's got a wife."

"It's bloody disgusting," said Ginger. He didn't alter the reasonable tone of his voice, nor did he look at her. He'd placed his hands on the edge of the table as if to steady himself.

She stood up and moved regretfully to the door. "I egged him on," she insisted. "It wasn't his fault. He was the innocent party." She didn't wait for Ginger to reply. She realized she'd made a mistake telling him about Edward and herself— he was far too narrow in his outlook to make allowances.

The woman in the hall was awake and massaging her ribs. By her side lay a large celluloid doll without clothes. "You," she called. "If Ginger's finished with you, make us a drink. I'm parched." She was grinning.

"I'm just about to put the kettle on," said Binny. She went through into the kitchen. She didn't feel at all sorry for the woman and was puzzled by this lack of compassion. She stepped over the still slumbering Harry and put the kettle on the stove. She took cups and a bottle of milk to the table. Alma sat hunched in a corner of the sofa, knees drawn up to her chin. Muriel lay face downwards, large legs thrust beyond Alma's shoulders, feet braced against the wall. "You're awake," said Binny.

"No," snapped Alma. "I always sleep with my eyes open." She was now perfectly sober and feeling belligerent.

"I've been upstairs talking to Ginger," Binny told her. "He's not at all menacing once you get through to him. I was terrified they'd done something to Edward. I learned quite a lot. He's going to tell us what he intends to do."

"You always were a rotten judge of character," said Alma. "He's weird. I wouldn't touch him with a barge pole."

"He's not weird," protested Binny. "He's not at all like Harry or that swine Widnes—"

Alma said she was being absurd. Widnes had acted in a brutal manner because he thought he'd been double-crossed. The woman asked for everything she got.

"You'd passed out," said Binny crossly. "He tried to strangle her."

"Well, he was annoyed, pet. You'd have done the same. There's nothing wrong with a bit of healthy anger. And Harry's harmless enough. He's a bit slow—"

"He wasn't slow smashing my lampshade," cried Binny. It was just like Alma to get the wrong end of the stick. It was useless discussing anything with her. "I ticked Ginger off about breaking the window," she said. "He was quite apologetic. I tried to get him to release Edward."

"You are funny," said Alma. "You worry over Teddy, but when you're together you never stop goading the poor man. The way you sulked when he mentioned buying aspirins for his wife. If looks could kill—"

Binny attempted to straighten the tablecloth but gave up. She couldn't trip backwards and forwards across the sleeping gunman on the floor. She wished Alma hadn't referred to Helen as "his wife"—it was illogical of her, she knew, but the possessive pronoun hurt. She said tearfully, "What will she do when she learns about Edward and me? She's bound to find out now, isn't she?"

"She knows already, darling. You and I would. Why do you keep thinking she's any different?"

"She doesn't know. Edward says—"

"Rubbish," snapped Alma. "She's probably been trailing him for months." She smiled suddenly. "Do you remember that time I thought

148

Frank was carrying on with a girl at the office? You were useless. You kept saying please God don't let's find him."

"I know," said Binny. She hadn't enjoyed the incident—following Frank all over London in the passenger seat of Alma's little car, shooting through traffic lights, Alma driving with one hand and swigging whisky out of a bottle with the other. People looked down on them from buses. Binny was terrified they might actually spot Frank and he would hurl himself across the bonnet of the car. He had a very nasty temper. Alma made her wear a wig from Woolworths and sunglasses. They went into the most unlikely places in search of him—the crypt of St. Paul's, under the arches of the embankment. "For God's sake," Binny had argued, clutching her horrendous wig in the wind and standing ankle deep in filth, "he's supposed to be courting, not doing away with her." In the end they sat for three hours outside the house of Frank's auntie in Battersea, in case he was using the place as a rendezvous.

"I wish he'd run off with some woman now," said Alma. "I'd be glad to get him off my hands. I hid the clock to annoy him before I came out. How's the poor sod going to get up for work?"

"Do you think the neighbors will take in the children?" asked Binny.

"Not if they've any sense, darling. I don't suppose Victor will notice I'm not there. Not until the food runs out." Alma swung her feet on to the carpet and stood upright in the gloom. She fretted over the state of her dress and her hair. "I look as if I've been down a coal mine," she accused. "What on earth did you do to me when I was so ill?"

Binny ignored her and went through to make the pot of tea. She'd noticed there were splinters of light bulb among the bread crumbs on the table. She wondered if she dared make Widnes a cheese-and-glass sandwich. When she returned to the table, Alma was standing leaning against the wall talking to the wallpaper. "This is Alma Waterhouse calling, pet," she said. "Will you please tell Frank the alarm clock's in the kitchen cupboard. Repeat . . . in the kitchen cupboard. Thank you very much." She looked defiantly at Binny. "Well, he'll be looking all over for it, darling."

Binny asked Alma to take the woman in the hall a cup of tea. She didn't know what to do about the others. She stood at the open door and called brightly, "Tea up." Scuttling back into the room, fearful lest Harry should wake in alarm and point a gun at her, she sat down at the table. She waited. Alma came back holding a doll in her arms.

"How does she seem?" asked Binny.

"She's very butch, pet. She's got hair on her knuckles." Alma looked at the disordered room. "Isn't it funny, not having to do anything? We're not expected to clear this up, there's no meals to prepare, no beds to make. It's hardly likely we'll be asked to go shopping. People pay good money for this sort of life at holiday camps."

"I hate mess," said Binny. "It makes me sick."

"The children must feel like this all the time," Alma remarked. "Never expected to do anything, sitting in squalor, ordered about. It's very restful." She gazed compassionately at the naked doll in her arms. "Poor wee thing," she crooned. "It'll catch its death of cold. Did I ever tell you about my brother taking his trousers off in Marks and Spencers?"

"Several times," said Binny. "Ginger's got a brother, you know. He's been in Walton jail. But Ginger's never been in prison. So he says."

"He's been in a bank though, darling," Alma said. She rocked the ugly doll. "I peeped in the pram. It's full of five pound notes wrapped in a woolly blanket."

Muriel reared her head above the arm of the sofa. Neck wobbling, staring at Alma like a child waking from a bad dream, she opened her mouth and screamed.

14

When Edward was brought into the kitchen he embraced Binny and kissed her hair. He didn't care who was watching. "Little one," he murmured into her ear, stroking her back with the stem of his pipe. "I'm sorry." He meant all the times he'd not been able to be with her. Lying curled in the empty bath and hearing that animal shriek of terror in the room along the hall, he had felt his heart break into pieces. He couldn't bear to think of her afraid and alone. She was his responsibility. Even though he now understood it was Simpson's wife who had screamed, he clutched Binny's hand and vowed not to leave her. He was strengthened in his resolve by the growing conviction that the gunmen were decent chaps after all. They had allowed him to wash and make himself more comfortable. Widnes had encouraged Simpson to dab mercurochrome, found in the bathroom cupboard, on his damaged ankle bone. And now they were all gathered in the front room, candles lit in milk bottles, enjoying a cup of tea and slices of bread and cheese. Ginger even suggested it would be a pity not to finish the wine. He and his men wouldn't themselves partake—a further point, Edward felt, in their favor —because they needed their wits about them for the morning siege. Only Alma Waterhouse took advantage of the offer. It was true Muriel sat shuddering over a measure of sherry, but that was medicinal and purely to calm her nerves. Simpson wasn't awfully good at coping with his wife in her present state of mind. He spoke brusquely to her once or twice and told her to pull herself together. He made excuses to Edward. "She's been overdoing it lately," he muttered. "Housework, that sort of thing. Mowing the lawn, shifting the furniture. Don't know what's got into her." Edward found her behavior perfectly justifiable. In the same situation Helen would be lying on the floor crying, or else abusing him for their predicament. He couldn't help admiring Alma, sitting there in her shiny red frock, tossing back the wine and smiling affectionately around the table. There was quite a festive atmosphere in the room, with the candles flickering and the shadow of the pink carnations frilly upon the wall. The barrels of guns leapt like spiked leaves among the flowers.

To everyone's embarrassment Ginger brought up the fact that Edward was a married man. "I can't hold myself responsible for your morals," he told him. "That's your lark, not mine. I don't hold with you deceiving your missus, but I'm sorry if we've added to your difficulties."

"My dear fellow," cried Edward, growing red in the face. "It couldn't be helped. You weren't to know."

"Nobody asked you to be here," flashed Binny.

"Stop it,' admonished Alma. She tapped Binny's flushed face with her glass. "You're at it again."

Moved, Edward made a little speech. "I'm not saying my way of life isn't despicable, but I mean it sincerely when I say how glad I am to be at Binny's side during this ordeal." He glanced emotionally at her and cleared his throat. "I wouldn't like`you to be alone."

He was astonished at his declaration in front of so many witnesses. Not that it mattered any longer, and even if it had Helen wasn't in the habit of consorting with the criminal classes; but still his bravery and indiscretion cheered him. He said delightedly, "Not that it's much of an ordeal at the moment. I think we all understand one another well enough."

"God Almighty," murmured Simpson.

The gunmen sipped their tea and said nothing.

"The reason I'm alone, as you put it," remarked Binny resentfully, "is because society's altered. If this was forty years ago, I'd have my husband by my side. He wouldn't have run off with that woman from the telephone exchange. My mother and father stayed together, and they didn't like each other. It's only a question of fashions changing."

Edward was sure Binny had told him her husband had deserted her for an actress or a model of some sort. Perhaps she had been the speaking clock at one time. "I've stayed with my family," he said gently. He was trying to give Binny hope, show her the world wasn't all bad. "Some of us have retained the old standards."

"My dad didn't have a woman on the side," said Binny.

"What do you intend to do in the morning?" asked Simpson. "How long do you think this can go on?"

"That depends," said Ginger.

"On what?" demanded Simpson aggressively. "Famine, disease, sudden death? That woman in the hall needs a doctor. Ribs are tricky things. She could have perforated a lung."

Widnes sniggered.

"Why don't you let all the women go?" persisted Simpson. In the candlelight his round face was stern and resolute. Already the stubble of a beard was appearing along his cheek bones and his upper lip. "My wife's in a pretty poor state.

You'll have to answer for the consequences."

"We'll do that," said Ginger drily. "There's things we're not going to tell you, things they're piecing together at the moment." He jerked his head in the direction of the shutters.

"Are you trying to obtain money?" asked Edward. "Ransom money?"

"Not that," Ginger said. "We just need to get away."

"I've every sympathy," Edward told him. "It must be hell on earth. I don't mind telling you I'd have gone under. One day confined to bed with a cold and I'm bored silly."

"Anybody mind if I have a slash?" asked Simpson. He stood up and moved casually to the door, taking his cup with him.

"You could tell them you wanted an airplane, pet," Alma said to Ginger. "They'd have to give you one. You could make for Rio."

"If I was you," advised Edward, "I'd behave with great diplomacy. You mustn't antagonize the authorities. You should proceed with cunning. How would it be if I composed a letter for you, outlining your demands, etc.? It would impress them, you know."

"He's awfully good at writing letters," conceded Binny.

Widnes was turned toward the back window, listening.

"Something along these lines," began Edward. "It is beneficial to all concerned that this—"

"Belt up," cried Widnes violently.

Distinctly they heard the scrape of a bolt being drawn, the sound of a door banging against a distant wall.

The men stampeded from the room. There were shouts and the splintering of wood as a door was kicked inwards.

"Oh God," moaned Binny.

"Don't worry, don't worry," soothed Edward, unable to rise from his chair. "They won't do anything. The guns aren't loaded. Nothing will happen."

He was still babbling in this demented fashion when a deafening report drowned his words. The ensuing silence lasted for several seconds. Then Harry was in the room, standing just inside the doorway of the kitchen.

"Out," he ordered, speaking to Edward.

His heart leaping in his breast, Edward stumbled down the hall and into the bathroom. The jamb of the door hung askew from the wall. He was reminded of Binny's description of middle age, of the second half of the match in progress. He imagined the whistle had already gone. God was waiting in the yard. Trembling in every limb, he was thrust through the garden door and on to the veranda.

"Fetch him," hissed Ginger. "Get the bugger up here."

Like an obliging dog retrieving a stick, Edward descended the steps. He was buffeted by the wind.

Branches of trees rocked against the sky. The embedded glass on the back wall sparkled under a hurtling moon. I shall drown, Edward thought; I shall be dashed to pieces on the rocks. Simpson was lying at the foot of the steps, clutching the hose attachment of a hoover to his chest. He was swearing like a midshipman.

"Get up," said Edward. "For Christ's sake, get up." He gripped Simpson under the armpits and tried to lift him.

"Piss off," cried Simpson.

"Your wife," entreated Edward. "Think of your wife. Miriam needs you."

"Fuck Miriam," moaned Simpson.

They struggled over possession of the hoover. The rubber hose wrapped itself about Edward's knees. Desperately he heaved Simpson on to his feet. He didn't care if the man was bleeding to death and shouldn't be moved; they were standing up there, the three gunmen, urging him to hurry. Half carrying, half dragging Simpson, Edward manhandled him up the steps and on to the veranda. Both men lay stranded on their bellies, gasping for breath. Roughly they were hauled inside the bathroom.

"The back wall's swarming with the bastards," panted Ginger.

Simpson struggled to his knees. He looked down appalled at the front of his shirt. An enormous red stain spread from his shoulder to his waist.

"I never hit you," cried Widnes. "You weren't even in sight." He bent over Simpson and examined his head. "It's nothing," he said at last, reaching for the mercurochrome bottle that still stood on the washstand. He had fired at the wall; a fragment of brick had ricocheted across the yard and sliced the lobe of Simpson's ear.

Simpson bled like a pig. He hadn't known his body could contain so much blood. He imagined he was growing paler with each drop that drained away.

"It needs more than mercurochrome," said Edward. He himself felt he needed a heart transplant. More dead than alive, spattered with Simpson's blood, he sat on the edge of the bath and fought for breath.

It was ten to four by his watch.

15

Everyone's sympathy lay with the gunmen. They had intimated what might happen if anybody tried to escape. What were they supposed to do under the circumstances? They couldn't let people run away in all directions. And Simpson hadn't been shot, merely lacerated by a portion of flying brick.

"Teddy did warn you," said Alma, winding a length of cotton sheeting about Simpson's head. "But you wouldn't be told."

"They'll think he's dead," Binny said. "They'll have sent for reinforcements."

Muriel sat passively on the sofa, staring at the shuttered windows. Apart from glancing at her husband and frowning at his discolored shirt, she took no interest in his condition.

"You said there was only a rabbit hutch," fumed Simpson. "Why do you keep a hoover in the garden?"

"You are extravagant, darling," said Alma reproachfully. "There was no need to throw it out just because it hadn't a plug."

Edward was worried lest the police would misunderstand what had occurred in the yard. It was important for them all that the friendly relationship built up over the last few hours should be maintained. "Couldn't I explain?" he asked Ginger. "You know, call out to the police? Let them know the position?"

"What good will it do?" Ginger said.

"Well, don't you see, now that they think you're dangerous men, their attitude will be different. They won't trust you. They might even place sharp-shooters on the roof ready to pick you off when you pass the windows."

"They're there already," said Harry.

"This isn't Chicago," protested Edward. "I do think you should follow my advice."

After some discussion Edward tied his handkerchief to the head of the sweeping brush and approached the back window. Binny had suggested he appear on the balcony, but he worried in case Helen might be out there in the street. The words would have died on his lips.

It took quite some time to wrench up the window. Holding a furled newspaper to his mouth and thrusting the broom into the night, Edward shouted: "This is a hostage speaking. I am a hostage." Behind him, Alma giggled. "The gun shot you heard was a misunderstanding. We are unhurt. Nobody has been shot. We are all well and cheerful."

"Speak for yourself," muttered Simpson, clutching his bandaged ear.

"Mention your shirt," said Binny. "You're covered in blood."

"My shirt," shouted Edward, "Is not what it seems." He waited. There was no reply from the moonlit garden.

"They'll think you're under duress," whispered Binny. "They probably think there's a gun in your back."

Ginger slammed down the window.

Edward wasn't satisfied. He felt it wasn't enough to say they were unhurt—they should be seen to be unharmed. He took Ginger to one side and told him it might be for the best if they were all observed together, chatting normally.

"Chatting?" said Ginger.

"You know, informally. No sign of strain. What about upstairs?"

"There's no space," said Ginger. "You can't go up there. We've put the table in front of the windows." He was overwhelmed by Edward. He didn't know how to check him.

"The table," cried Edward. "That's perfect. Of course. It's bound to put their minds at rest."

Powerless to dampen his enthusiasm, the gunmen accompanied Edward as he cajoled his troupe up the stairs. Muriel stayed on the sofa.

They heaved the table on to its legs. Harry and Widnes watched from the doorway. Ginger sat on the stairs smoking a cigarette.

Edward urged Simpson to remove his bandage.

"Leave me alone," shouted Simpson furiously. He lashed out at Edward with his fist.

Offended, Edward backed away. The man's pain had turned him into an animal. "He's got money troubles," he murmured to Binny. "He's up to his eyes in debt." He supposed at a distance the blood on Simpson's shirt might be taken for some kind of pattern.

"We've got paddles," said Binny, fetching them from under the bed. "But there isn't a ball."

"Never mind," cried Edward. "It won't be seen." Like an impresario he arranged the setting. "Lights," he called.

The gunmen shuffled backwards on to the landing. Alma, her arms about Simpson's waist, supported him at the table. He blinked in the light. A green paddle was shoved into his hand.

"Laugh," ordered Edward. "Look as if you're enjoying yourselves." He served an imaginary ball across the net. He ducked, slammed, made a little leap in the air.

"He's very good," observed Alma, watching the game from beneath Simpson's armpit.

For almost a minute Simpson remained

propped at the table, mesmerized by his opponent's play. Then, stamping his foot in a tantrum, he tore free from Alma's embrace and hurled his paddle across the room.

"What a bad sport!" chided Alma, avoiding his flailing arms.

"Lights off," shouted Edward. Exhausted, he led the way onto the landing.

"You," said Ginger, tapping Binny on the shoulder, "I want a word."

Going downstairs, Edward felt there was nothing more he could do. He hoped the newspaper reports wouldn't distort the scene at the ping-pong table. He wanted Helen to read that he was alive and well, not having the time of his life. He wondered if he hadn't overdone the laughter.

16

Preceding Ginger into the bedroom, Binny was already composing in her head sentences she would repeat later to Edward and the others. I don't really know myself why he chose to confide his plans to me. Perhaps I remind him of someone . . . he has a sister, you know. Mind you, we hit it off right from the beginning. Perhaps it's a little fanciful, but I had the feeling we were on the same wave-length. It happens sometimes—

"Over there," said Ginger.

She looked across the room. He was staring at the divan bed shoved against the far wall.

"Hurry up," he said.

She wasn't sure if she'd understood him. They'd been such pals.

"Get your drawers off," he urged.

She was astounded. She said, "Don't be silly."

He took hold of her arm and squeezed it tightly. "Do as you're told."

She sat down on the bed and began to unzip the side of her dress. She was showing all her teeth and grinning in the near darkness. She felt ridiculous. It would have been better if he'd threatened her with a gun or smashed her across the face instead of pinching her arm in that spiteful fashion.

"No," he said sharply. "I don't want you with nothing on. Only take your stockings off."

She thought he was very old-fashioned. She hadn't worn stocking for years. Swivelling round on the bed so that her back was to him, she began to wriggle out of her tights. She hoped her feet didn't smell. Just taking her shoes off made her feel suddenly very tired and shaky. It was the cleaning she'd done in the morning—or was it yesterday? Not to mention the shopping, the cooking, rowing with the children. All that energy, all that locomotion, hour after hour after hour—

"Lie down," he ordered.

She lay flat and hoped he wouldn't strangle her. It didn't seem very likely, not with everybody sitting downstairs, talking and making jokes. She distinctly heard the trill of Alma's laughter. If he put his hands round her throat, once she was sure he really meant to harm her, she would jab him in the crotch with her knee. She couldn't do it immediately because his hands weren't anywhere near her neck and she had to give him the benefit of the doubt. She wasn't sure whether you could kill somebody by banging them there. She would rather die than act too hastily.

"Do you want to feel my chest?" she said. She was showing him she was uninhibited and matter of fact about the whole business. He needn't worry that she would throw hysterics or start imagining that he was madly in love with her. She was a woman of the world.

"Keep quiet," he said. "I can't abide tits."

The neck of his woolly jumper smelled of after-shave; he was resting the point of his chin on her forehead. She moved, and for an instant his mouth brushed hers. He jerked his head away. He didn't touch her at all; he just slipped inside.

She kept thinking of Lawrence of Arabia feeling ashamed at being done so easily. It hadn't made it very clear in the film what had happened to him. He merely came out of the man's tent looking a bit po-faced and walked off into the desert in a funny stiff way as if he'd been on a horse all his life. She wouldn't have known what it meant except somebody told her the following day. But it was understandable really, him being excited and ready for it. It wasn't anything to do with wanting it—the rudeness of the whole thing accomplished the necessary lubrication. The divan was awfully uncomfortable. When Harry had tugged the sheet from the bed he'd messed up the blankets. There was something digging into her back and she wriggled.

"Stop that," said Ginger.

"I'm sorry," she said.

She supposed she was being raped. One huge tear gathered in her left eye and rolled down her cheek. She wasn't feeling hurt or humiliated—he didn't do anything dirty or unusual. He wasn't stubbing cigarettes out on her despised breasts or swinging from the chandelier, member pointed like a dagger. It was unreal, of no account. That's why she cried—though she wondered why it was only in one eye. It would be better not to mention any of this to a soul, not even under torture. Unless she had bruises to show for it or a nervous breakdown, people would have doubts. It was like when small children were molested on the way back from sweet shops. However sympathetic one felt towards the distraught parents, there were always those reservations. Why was the child out at that time of night? What was she doing on her own? It was dreadful, but blame was apportioned.

Ginger was clutching her head and muttering one word over and over. She couldn't be sure, because his fingers were stuffed in her ears, but it sounded like steak, steak, steak. It was funny the way persons behaved at certain times. During the war, when bombs were dropping or ships were going down, people coupled. Men grunted in the blackout.

She wasn't even young enough, she realized when Ginger rolled off her, to feel sorry for herself. It hadn't mattered that much. He was an ineffectual young man.

He jumped up almost at once and fastened his trousers; he stood smoothing the hair back from his forehead.

"Everything worked perfect," he said. "Those mates of mine did everything right, nobody got hurt. We got the bloke at the bank by the short and curlies. The kids went home. They'll know that by now. We rang up on the dot, like we said —on the bleeding dot."

"My son," Binny said, "wants a motorbike. I shan't let him have one."

"We all left at the same time. Geoff went off down the back of Lemon Street. We weren't half feeling chuffed. He was meant to come up by the cinema and down past the pet shop. When we couldn't spot him we went round in circles."

"I nearly bought a puppy there," said Binny. "Alison wanted one. He was lovely—he had a little fat tummy. It's quite an expense, you know. They have to have injections for 'flu and things."

"We were singing in the taxi. Widnes was bouncing up and down like a budgie on a perch."

Binny sat up and felt with her toes for the discarded tights. "Do you know, I passed there one

169

night and there were rats running over the floor.
I expect they were drawn by the birdseed. There
was one sitting in a cage with a canary. Honestly.
The poor thing was turned the other way with its
head on its wing, pretending it wasn't happening."

"Get up," said Ginger. "You go downstairs
first. You let out one word and I'll bust that fat
bloke's nose."

It wasn't light but the birds were singing. It
was like being in the country. It had been happening forever, thought Binny, nights passing, dawn
coming. All over the city people were lying in
bed, either in pairs or alone. In the park, two
streets away, grass beaded with dew, health fiends
ran in track suits along the cinder paths, hurdling
squirrels. Organized people had the breakfast
table ready laid.

17

It was worse in the morning. More sordid. Harry opened the shutters a fraction and let in daylight. There were plates of congealed food, broken glass, clothing strewn about the room. Even the pink carnations seemed blowsy. Simpson lay like a road casualty under the table; specks of dried blood freckled the knuckles of his outflung hand.

Harry marched them to the bathroom. They stood patiently in the passage awaiting their turn. Binny was concerned that her son's bicycle was badly damaged.

"He'll be so angry," she told Edward, fingering the bent spokes of the rear wheel. "He loves his bike."

"It doesn't matter," said Edward gently. "We'll

buy him a new one." He looked terrible and appeared to be itching all over. He had run out of tobacco and constantly rummaged in the pockets of his wrinkled suit, hoping for a miracle.

I've turned him into an incontinent tramp, thought Binny, regarding his unshaven face, puffy above a shirt collar rusted with Simpson's blood.

Muriel's appearance, despite her dishevelled clothes, was wholesome. She had slept longer than any of them and her naturally wavy hair and plump cheeks were an advantage. Her mouth, rubbed free of scarlet lipstick, curved full and rosy.

"You do look rested," said Alma suspiciously. She herself, waxen-faced, eyes curiously exposed without her false lashes, waited corpselike in her satin dress. Her body, slender in the candle glow, had turned to skin and bone in the morning light.

Widnes stayed in the bathroom while they used the lavatory. He stood facing the yard with his hands over his ears. He hummed a tune. When it was Muriel's turn she ordered him from the room. He obeyed, lumbering down the passageway with his fair hair sticking up in tufts and his shoulders bowed.

Edward made tea. He helped Simpson to a chair and inspected his wound. He fetched warm water in a porridge bowl and tenderly swabbed the mutilated ear. "Does it hurt much?" he asked.

"Only when I laugh," said Simpson sarcastically. When he kissed Marcia, she had a habit of twining her fingers in his hair. Finding his hair scanty, she ended by caressing the lobe of his ear. He doubted if she was going to bother in the future. Seeing his creased and ravaged countenance in the bathroom mirror he had realized his dancing days were over. To hell with Marcia, with her flat mates, her playmates, her unknown men answering the telephone. Women were used to men losing their hair. They didn't expect ears to recede as well; he wasn't Van Gogh. Touched by Edward's obvious concern, he said reluctantly: "Sorry about last night. I should have exercised a little more self-control. I must say, I was in the most damnable pain."

"My dear chap," cried Edward. "Don't say another word."

Simpson had no intention of doing so. He was embarrassed at recalling the woman sitting in the hall with her back to the door. It would have been far more sensible if he'd made a break for it that way; one heave at her ankles and he'd have been down the steps in a jiffy.

There was no fraternization between the gunmen and their hostages while morning tea was drunk. They each stayed in separate halves of the room, rubbing their eyes and yawning.

Ginger, using the top of the fridge as a desk, was writing a letter. Earlier he had asked Binny for pen and paper and she'd torn the middle section out of Alison's spelling book and given it to him. He wanted a dictionary as well, but she couldn't find one.

Edward sat on the floor and leaned his head wearily against the radiator.

"Please forgive me," said Binny. She squatted earnestly in front of him, cupping her hands round a mug of tea. "I realize I've been selfish. I'll go and talk to Helen when it's all over. I'll make her see I'm not important."

"Shh," he said.

"I'll make her understand it was just a diddle on the side. It didn't mean a thing."

"But it does," he said. "You've never understood."

"Well," she said. "I'll make it all right. You'll see."

He searched his pockets again and fell back defeated. "I don't know that I want it to be all right," he said. "I see things now in a different perspective. I've been thinking about love—"

"Love?" she said, looking away from him in embarrassment.

"It was always a stumbling block as far as I was concerned . . . right from childhood. Of course, my father—"

"Shall I get you some more tea?" Binny asked.

"No," he said. "I don't want tea. What I felt for my father, my school, was quite normal. In the circumstances. Then later, after I'd suffered that shock, I used other emotions, but I thought it was the same thing. You see what I mean?"

"Well," Binny said dubiously. "It's not crystal clear."

"I met that rotter Muldoon, you know, a few years ago at some conference or other. He seemed to have shrunk. Do you know, he didn't remember me. It was quite genuine . . . his forgetfulness. And I'd thought of him for thirty years. Isn't it amazing?"

"Very," said Binny.

"He looked quite prosperous. Didn't look as if he'd been near a cricket pitch for years. I found myself apologizing because I'd drunk the last of the water in the jug. I'm always apologizing . . . doing my best. It's a symptom. I've read about it since."

"You've read a lot," Binny said.

"I mean one should apologize . . . I think courtesy is very important, but it can be carried too far. I don't see the harm in telling her I want to lead a different kind of life. Do you? She does have her meetings to fall back on. I don't honestly think she'd mind."

"Oh dear," said Binny. It was typical of Edward to start talking in these terms when she was filthy dirty and worn out and they might be shot at any moment. She thought of all the times she had leaned towards him over the dinner table in some restaurant and willed him to say something like this. He'd talked instead about old Witherspoon and old Carmichael, until the lovely feeling went from her heart and she sat stiff as a poker

175

looking down at the menu, unable to order artichokes or prawns or anything really special and
tasty, because she might choke on them with disappointment. They would have turned to ashes in
her mouth.

"Look," she said. "You're overwrought. When
all this is over you'll have to tell Helen the truth
and I promise you it will be all right. She'll forgive you. You needn't worry about me. I shall get
over it."

I was raped not so long ago, she could have told
him, and I hardly remember that.

"But I'd like to be with you," Edward said. "It
would be fun." He was staring at her full in the
face. For once he didn't notice the blotches on her
cheeks, the state of her hair. He needed someone.

"What about your garden?" she reminded him.
"You couldn't leave your roses. Imagine all those
little insects and things burrowing into the buds
and nobody there to spray them."

"I often think I want the roses," he said, "because I had them as a child. I wake in the night
thinking about that garden. I sit at the window
and watch the sun rise and imagine my father
walking through the dew with his gun under his
arm." He rubbed his eyes as though tired of
searching for that solitary figure in gum boots.
"They're my father's roses," he said. "In a manner of speaking."

"You should rest," Binny said.

"I don't need to rest," he protested. "I can't.

Everything's so real now. It's all so real."

She gathered he meant the presence of the gun-men, the disordered room, their imprisonment. For the life of her, she couldn't understand him —to her it was like a dream.

"Think of it this way," she said. "It all equals out. Take Simpson and Muriel. They're together and yet they're not. We're not together and yet we are." She touched his wrinkled cheek.

"I feel dreadful about poor Simpson," he said. "Simply dreadful. I should have watched him more carefully. I don't think we should blame Muriel too much. She's pretty highly strung, you know, and he doesn't confide in her as he ought."

"She's highly something," said Binny. She looked at Muriel sitting composedly in the arm-chair by the hearth, genteelly sipping her tea. Though for some reason she'd screamed at the sight of the doll, she hadn't made a sound when her husband entered covered in blood.

"He's in serious financial difficulties," Edward said. "I shouldn't tell you this, but he's terribly overdrawn at the bank—"

"He's overwhat?" Binny asked. She put her arms about Edward's neck and asked again. "He's what?"

"Shh," said Edward. He peeped over her shoul-der. Simpson was lying with his good ear to the cloth, face turned to the back window. "His busi-ness isn't going too well. He complains when Muriel goes to the hairdresser and so forth, but he never confides in her. I think it's frightfully wrong of him."

"Does he tell her about his women?" asked Binny. "Does she know about the V.D.?"

"Good Lord, no," said Edward, shocked.

Binny wrenched her arms from his neck and glared at him. "Oh yes," she said. "He should tell her about his money problems, shouldn't he? He ought to worry her silly over the bills and the mortgage, but he should keep his extramarital affairs to himself. Share his burdens but not his pleasures. You make me sick." She sprang to her feet and flounced through to the kitchen.

Ginger was leaning against the draining board. She shoved him out of the way and began noisily to slide the dishes into the sink.

18

Ginger switched on the wireless at midday to listen to the news.

"Don't touch it," warned Binny. "It won't go at all if you move it." The wireless was old and there was a lot of interference. Alma said it was like being in the underground, crowding round an illegal transmitter, waiting to hear Churchill's voice.

"Illegal?" questioned Edward. "In the tube station?"

"Shh," said Simpson, endeavoring to listen with one ear.

There was a report of an air disaster somewhere in Latin America and a fire in New York. Nearer home an M.P. had died and the two grandchildren of a bank manager in Camden had been held to ransom for seven hours while thieves coolly cashed checks totalling thousands of pounds.

"Why do they always say 'coolly'?" said Alma. "It's so silly. I bet they don't feel cool at all."

"I can't hear," complained Simpson. It was giving him a headache trying to make sense of the news reader's words. He wandered irritably up and down the room.

When the news was over Edward said they were obviously being very cagey. Rightly so.

"Who are?" demanded Simpson.

"The authorities," said Edward. "Didn't you listen?"

"I don't wear this for show," cried Simpson, touching the bandage wound about his head.

Ashamed of his stupidity, Edward repeated the news announcer's report. Armed men had entered a house in North London and were holding an unspecified number of women and children as hostages. No names were available as yet.

"I don't call that cagey," Simpson said crossly. "It's damned inaccurate."

"Fancy going in and out of a bank all day," said Binny, "cashing checks. I do think it's clever. Every time anyone queried the amounts I expect the poor manager just nodded his head."

"There's no sodding food," Harry said. He swung the fridge door violently on its hinges.

Apart from the half-pound of sausages there

wasn't anything to eat. No bread, butter or eggs. There weren't any tins of baked beans in the cupboard.

"I don't hold with bulk buying," Binny said defensively. "Take fruit. If I buy several pounds of fruit, the children give it to their friends. So I buy three oranges and three apples fresh every day and dole them out. It's more economical."

"There's no need to apologize," said Edward. "You're not running a cafeteria. If necessary we can ask for supplies. I believe it's quite usual." He began to write a list in the margin of his newspaper.

"My ear hurts," Simpson said peevishly. He waited for his wife to respond. She was mute. He couldn't imagine what was going on in her head. Not once had she mentioned the children.

He rose from the table and went to stand beside her. "Muriel," he said loudly. He prodded her leg with his bare toes. "Muriel—"

"Yes," she said.

"The girls?" he asked. "They'll be worried, won't they?"

She wouldn't answer.

"Did you tell them where we were going?"

"I may have," she said. "But they wouldn't have listened."

"Did you turn the kitchen light off?"

"Go away," she said.

He seized hold of her arm and shook her. He couldn't prove it, but he knew she was being deliberately provocative—it had nothing to do with their present situation. "It may be of little interest to you," he told her, "but I pay the electricity bills."

"You should see what they've done to your car,' she said. 'You'll need a new fender and a door."

He opened the shutters wider and stared into the little garden. The sun was shining on the privet hedge. He fetched a chair from the table and climbing upon it tried to see over the hedge into the street. "There's no cars out there," he said.

"Get away from that window," shouted Harry. He raised his fist threateningly.

Simpson closed the shutters and remained standing on the chair. "My car," he complained. "What's happened to my car?"

"They moved them all," said Ginger. "In the night. They've roped off the block."

"They rammed yours, George," Muriel said. "With a taxi. I saw them."

Simpson stepped down from the chair and leaned sluggishly against the fireplace; he yawned repeatedly. His wife sat a million miles from him, playing with a thread of cotton at the torn hem of her frock. He had always imagined that this sort of experience drew people closer together, made them nobler and more sensitive. He'd seen photographs of survivors of such dramas, and it had seemed to him that their eyes were tranquil with communal suffering. He glanced in the mirror and was unmoved by the frayed bandage tied in a small bow at the top of his balding head. He watched Ginger go to the kitchen door and turn to beckon Muriel.

"You," Ginger said. "I want a word with you."

Muriel tugged the thread from her dress and, rising, followed him into the hall.

"Oh God," said Binny.

Edward was struggling to compose a shopping list. He had pencilled the word "tobacco" several times along the edge of the newspaper. He couldn't think of anything else; he found it difficult to concentrate. He had always left the shopping to Helen. He hadn't thought of her for over two hours—he hadn't thought of anything save his need for tobacco. His father too had smoked a pipe. When he'd gone to bed at night he'd left it under a cushion for safety. During the war, when tobacco was rationed, he'd stuffed wood shavings into the bowl and smoked those.

Edward was just considering whether bread crumbs could be utilized when he was ordered by Harry to go through to the bathroom. At the door he tried to pat Binny's shoulder, but she wouldn't let him. It appeared she was still put out by his earlier conversation, though he'd supposed her reaction would have been one of joy. He thought he'd offered to leave his wife. He certainly remembered saying it would be fun. He kept seeing his father holding a leather pouch on his lap, dabbling with his fingers in the moist shreds of tobacco.

"I don't know why he puts up with you," said Alma. "You'll be wearing jack-boots next and trampling all over him."

"Be quiet," said Binny. "It's nothing to do with Edward." She was waiting to hear Muriel scream. She looked at Harry and wondered if she dare confide in him—but then, if Alma was right and he was a bit slow, he wouldn't understand what she meant until it was too late.

Ginger came back into the room and told her she was needed upstairs. She stared at him as though he had spoken in a foreign language. He hadn't been absent for more than five minutes.

"Piss off," he ordered.

When she'd gone he took hold of Simpson by the slack of his ruined shirt and warned him not to go near the shutters or the back window. "We'll only be in the passage," he said. "And this time we won't hit the bleeding wall."

Weakly, Simpson nodded. He blinked his eyes rapidly to hide his tears; he hadn't been bullied since kindergarten.

The men wheeled the pram into the hall and left Simpson alone with Alma. He clenched his fists, waiting for her inane chatter to begin. She remained in the kitchen for a moment pouring the last of the sherry into a glass. He couldn't really blame her for wanting a drink. Marcia could put away a fair amount of booze. She was probably thinking his failure to telephone her this morning was due to pique—women always thought of themselves first.

Alma came to the table, sat down, and placed the glass at his elbow. Simpson looked at her. She had a small thin mouth and large eyes brimming with friendliness. She nodded encouragingly. Reduced again to tears, he was forced to turn his head away. Struggling to control his voice, he said with difficulty, "Thank you."

"Would you mind if we didn't talk?" said Alma. "I'd like to read the newspaper."

19

Climbing the stairs, Binny imagined Ginger intended to abuse both Muriel and herself: either one after the other, or together, if that was possible. She couldn't bear the idea of seeing Muriel without her stockings. This time, she thought, I shall protest. He'll have to shoot me. It was easier to be brave in daylight.

Muriel was bent over the divan, straightening the rumpled bedclothes. The injured woman lay on her side, stripped to the waist, face turned to the wall. The soles of her feet were black with dirt.

"We need something to bind her ribs with," Muriel said. "She's in pain. Do you have any more sheets?"

"Yes," lied Binny. "But they're at the laundry."

"We'll use these," Muriel decided. She slipped the pillows from beneath the woman's shoulder and took them to the ping-pong table. Discarding the pillows, she began to rip the frail cotton covers with her teeth.

"Were you ever a nurse?" asked Binny. She herself was hopeless in the sick room. The slightest cough or clearing of the patient's throat convinced her that the grim reaper was at hand.

Muriel said she'd done a first aid course at the Institute, two or three years ago. "I only did it to get out of the house," she explained. "Then later I used it as an excuse."

"I don't much like going out of the house," said Binny. "I do sometimes when Edward takes me to dinner, but not otherwise." She wondered if this was the moment to ask Muriel what she thought of Helen. She didn't think the two women were terribly friendly—Muriel hadn't once mentioned Helen during dinner—though perhaps she was just being tactful. Binny longed to hear that Helen was overweight or common or needed to wear a wig. "I didn't mean to interfere in their marriage," she said. "If he hadn't come to dinner she would never have known. I'd have given him up in the end."

"The third week," Muriel said, laying the strips of cotton in neat rows upon the green table, "we stopped sitting in front of the blackboard and did practical work. A man had fallen off a ladder and we attended to him."

"I'd have run the other way," admitted Binny. "I couldn't have gone near him."

"He hadn't really fallen off a ladder," Muriel said. "There were possible internal injuries and multiple fractures on both legs—"

"Good Heavens."

"I was given his right leg. I put on splints. The following week he treated me for burns. We met secretly for twelve months."

After a moment's silence, Binny asked: "What happened? Did Simpson find out?"

"We wanted somewhere to go. Once we went into a field, but it wasn't very satisfactory. I asked a woman friend of mine if we could use her house one afternoon. We'd been at school together. She'd met X and she said he was a fine man—we could have the house any time we wanted. We were always good chums at school. She even offered to have a key cut for me. Her husband was dead, you see, and she went out to work."

"What a nice woman," said Binny. She sensed some tragedy was about to be disclosed.

"When I told X he was delighted. It was Thursday and I'd been to the hairdresser. It rained and rained. We'd decided beforehand that it would be more exciting if I arrived first and waited for him like a wife . . . I'd let him in. It would be more like our own home—"

"Actually," objected Binny, "he'd have his key

if it was home." She could have bitten her tongue for putting her thoughts into words. Muriel had closed her eyes and was gripping the edge of the table.

She said: "I waited for hours. He didn't come. I never heard from him again."

Binny picked up the rags of cotton and wound them round her wrist; they weren't long enough to bind anybody's chest. "Perhaps he was run over," she said finally. She prayed he had been. How Muriel had suffered—waiting at a window for the kiss of life and recalling, while listening for the sound of Mr. X's footsteps squelching up the path, those nursing nights they'd swabbed and cleaned and tended imaginary wounds.

"I wore this dress," said Muriel.

Binny looked out into the street and saw a large crowd gathered behind a barrier on the corner; she almost waved. A television camera, angled on the roof of a van, was pointing directly at the house. She hoped the eggshells wouldn't show up in the bedraggled hedge. As she watched, craning for a glimpse of Lucy or Gregory, a door opened in the flats opposite. Draped in a travelling rug, Mrs. Papastavrou advanced to the balcony railings. One long high-pitched wail echoed along the street before several policemen leapt from other doorways and hustled her inside.

She's made a mistake, thought Binny. It can't be half-past six.

Behind her, the injured woman groaned. Leaving Muriel lost in nightmares at the table, Binny took a pillow to the divan; she was bending down to slip it into place when the woman groaned again, and uncurling herself from that fetal position against the wall lay flat on her back in the bed. She was a man.

20

They didn't see the house or the street on television after all. Something had gone wrong with the set.

"You do have trouble with your plugs, pet," said Alma, disappointed. She was hoping that Frank might have been interviewed and that he would have said what a wonderful wife and mother she was. It wasn't very likely, but then appearing on television did peculiar things to people.

Edward was brought from the bathroom at seven o'clock. He couldn't help remembering the night before when they'd eaten bread and cheese by candlelight. Binny said it was today, but he found it hard to believe. He had gone twelve hours without tobacco and was feeling both edgy and depressed. Simpson told him that his name hadn't actually been mentioned on the radio, but he'd been referred to as a prominent accountant.

"They mentioned Simpson's name," Alma told him. "They'd appealed for any information, and a woman came forward and said he'd telephoned her earlier in the evening." She beamed at Simpson proudly; she felt he was something of a celebrity.

"It's all nonsense," Simpson said wearily. "They get everything wrong." He didn't know why he was bothering to deny it—they could have said he was a notorious mass-murderer and Muriel wouldn't have noticed.

Ginger informed them that they were moving out before midnight. He'd taken a suitcase from the upstairs room and now sat with it firmly gripped between his knees. "Everybody hold on," he said. "And do as you're told."

"Moving out?" asked Edward, bewildered. "Where are we going?"

"Not you, Fatso," said Ginger. "Us and one of the women. Maybe two of them."

Edward didn't believe him; they were obviously bluffing. "I haven't written my letter," he told Simpson.

"When we go," Ginger said. "You and Curly Tops here will help Geoff into the cab. We'll follow with the women."

"Geoff?" said Edward. He noticed there was a packet of American cigarettes in the top pocket of Ginger's leather jacket. He was too proud to ask for one.

"That suitcase," whispered Simpson. "They must have stolen things from various parts of the house."

"There's nothing worth stealing," Edward said.

He roamed the kitchen, searching feverishly in the cupboard and the fridge for something to eat. The sausages had disappeared. He could make little sense of Binny's ramblings about the man upstairs being a woman. There were three potatoes in the vegetable rack, but he knew that if he cooked them they'd have to be shared out.

"She isn't a woman," said Binny. "She's a man. She's got hairs on her chest. Why don't you listen?"

"I'm so damned hungry," he complained miserably. "Can't you think where you put that pudding you lost?"

"It's in a shopping bag," said Binny. "That's all I know." She stared at him accusingly. "You're not worried about them taking me with them, are you? You couldn't care less."

"They're not going anywhere," said Edward distractedly. "Why don't you have a store cupboard?"

"She was in the bank this afternoon. Yesterday.

She smiled at me and I just knew there was something odd. She was looking me up and down like a man."

"Out of my way," said Edward. Binny was holding on to his arm and hampering his search. "Please stop getting under my feet."

She let go of him and stepped backwards to the sink.

"Don't," he pleaded, irritated by her pathetic expression. "Please forgive me. I'm so hungry." He put his arms round her and patted her back. Over her bowed head his eyes restlessly sought the shopping bag.

Binny said: "You promised we'd be together. Did you mean it?"

"Well," he said awkwardly. "I may have spoken out of turn. One does, you know."

"Does one?" she said contemptuously. Still, she remained in his embrace. "I thought you didn't care about the roses . . . you just wanted me."

"I do, I do," he murmured inadequately. "But not at this moment. I really can't think of anything, feeling the way I do." He propped her against the sink and peered in the corner beside the fridge. "It's all right for you," he grumbled. "You're not used to four-course lunches every day." He was disgusted to see small insects crawling in the cracks between the floorboards and the wall. "You really should clean this up. It's dreadfully unhygienic." He was shifting the fridge on its base, eager to uncover some verminous nest.

He saw a plastic bag wedged against the baseboard. "I've found it," he cried delightedly. He was astonished at the weight of the pudding. Parting the handles, he lifted out the silver balls. He set them on the window ledge. "I thought you meant a pie," he said. He could have wept with disappointment.

"All you think about," said Binny, "is your stomach or your roses. Or your precious wife. Nothing else matters. You don't know how the other half lives."

He frowned. "I never said she was precious. Certainly not in your hearing."

"I've been raped," said Binny.

He found he was smiling; he couldn't help it.

"By him," Binny said. She looked in the direction of the other room.

He saw Simpson slumped in the armchair with the absurd bow on his head.

"You're disgusting," she said. "You think it's a joke."

He moved to hold her, to comfort her.

"Don't come near me," she warned. "I don't know how I ever let you touch me. I'd need gloves to come near you."

Troubled, he tried to concentrate. He stared at the silver-coated apples on the windowsill; he was dazzled by sunlight. His father's hand, hidden in a leather glove, was raised to strike. Muldoon had split on him. He was a disgrace . . . not fit to mix with decent folk . . . I'm ashamed . . . I shan't forgive you. . . . The lovely shining badge skittered across a polished table. The field stretched green and sweet-smelling to the boundary line. That rotter Jonas, clothed in white, stood in the slips shielding his eyes from the glare of the sun . . .

Taking up an apple from the ledge, Edward rubbed it along his groin and, raising his arm, bowled from the shoulder at Simpson's head.

He missed. The apple smashed against the shutters, the silver paper unravelled and the fruit slid downwards, slimy on the woodwork. It plopped on to the carpet.

21

At ten o'clock Ginger ordered Edward and Simpson to help Geoff downstairs. Muriel said it would be far better if one of them carried him slung against their back like a baby in a shawl. That way it wouldn't hurt him so much.

"I can't do anything of that nature," said Simpson curtly. "I'd fall." He didn't relish the injured woman clutching his throbbing ear. Let Freeman do it. The damn fool seemed to have enough surplus energy—hurling things about the room in that irresponsible way when they were going to be released at any moment. His aim was ludicrous.

Edward experienced great difficulty in helping the woman down the stairs and into the hall. He couldn't think of her as a man. He didn't like to grasp her under the armpits in case he touched her breasts. When he dumped her on the floor by the front door he averted his eyes from her exposed thigh. He had dreams of telling Simpson to take his account elsewhere, and then of writing anonymously to the Inland Revenue accusing him of tax evasion.

The gunmen found a ladies' razor in the bathroom and shaved themselves. Clothes brushed and hair freshly combed, they waited for the police to knock at the door.

"It's all nonsense," Edward confided to Alma. "They can't possibly have arranged it."

"They did, pet," said Alma. "When you were in the bathroom. They used the telephohe." She'd asked Ginger twice who he intended to take with him, but he'd refused to answer. She wouldn't have minded being chosen; she was quite certain they'd be stopped by road blocks once they reached the open road. She wondered if her message about the alarm clock had got through. If it hadn't, it was possible that Frank and Victor were still fast asleep. If she went as a travelling hostage it would give them more time to wake up, and then none of her ordeal would be wasted. "Doesn't he look as if he's going on his holidays?" she said, beaming at Ginger, spruce in his chair, Binny's suitcase safe between his knees.

22

Some minutes after eleven o'clock, Ginger flung
the shutters wide; the broken window let in the
night air. They heard vehicles, voices in the
street. The women rose in agitation and touched
their tousled hair, smoothed their dresses.

"This is how it's going to be," said Ginger.
"And I don't want no mistakes." He stood Harry
and Widnes shoulder to shoulder in the center of
the room. He placed Edward in front of them,
facing outwards. He told Simpson and the
women to form a circle round the three in the
middle.

"Ring-a-ring-o'-roses," he shouted. "Link up."

Simpson was appalled to find he was holding
hands with Ginger. He tried to move places, but

the gunman held his fingers in a vice.

"Not so close," Ginger ordered. "Spread yourselves out."

"Why are we guarding Teddy, pet?" asked Alma.

"He's me," said Ginger. "He's standing in for me, isn't he? Right. We move down the hall like this and then on to the step. Nobody lets go. Anybody gets clever and I'll blow their head off. It doesn't matter now—there's a whole bloody army out there. We get to the car—"

"Holding hands?" said Edward. "Who's going to open the door?"

"When we reach the car, you and him"—Ginger stabbed his finger at Simpson and Edward—"you stay in the road and keep Harry in the middle. Then you go back into the house and get Geoff out of the bathroom."

"I can't remember all this," said Edward testily. "I've had very little sleep."

"Listen," Ginger said. "You and him don't get into—"

A voice, magnified nasally by a loud speaker, called from the street:

"Attention. Attention. Proceed to car, registration number OBY 439N, cream Cortina, stationed in middle of road. Engine running, rear left hand door open. Repeat, proceed to car—"

For an instant nobody moved. Then Ginger, breaking the chain of hands, went into the passage. "I'm warning you," he shouted. "Keep still."

A loud knocking began.

Ginger returned, pushing the pram ahead of him. He sent it free-wheeling toward the fridge. "I'm warning you," he repeated. "Hold hands."

Tottering backwards, the unwieldly circle oozed into the hall. The passage was so narrow they were pressed to each other like lovers. Glass crunched underfoot.

"You've forgotten your piggy bank, you know," said Alma, face to face with Widnes.

The exodus was halted while the suitcase was fetched from the kitchen. Cursing, Ginger thrust himself into the center of the scrum and, leaning across Harry's shoulder, tugged at the front door.

The whole world blazed with light. Concentrating on keeping the ring intact they flowed raggedly down the steps. They passed the hedge and jiggled out on to the pavement. One huge intake of breath, like a vast sigh, rose from the crowd on the corner.

Startled, the outer circle faltered, and seeing those massed figures not a hundred yards away felt a surge of pity for themselves. How kind they are, thought Binny, blinded by tears. They care about us.

Reaching the car, the group disintegrated. Widnes and Ginger thrust the three women into the interior of the Cortina and scrambled after them. Ginger, hampered by the bulky suitcase, crawled over the front seat and sat at the wheel. Mindful of their instructions, Edward and Simpson, with Harry in the middle, skipped sideways up the path again in a desperate barn-dance to the door.

Several minutes elapsed before the men reappeared. Harry carried Geoff on his back—one leg in a torn stocking dangled above the gutter. Widnes opened the far door of the car and shoved Muriel and Alma into the road. The women stood undecided.

I knew it would be me, thought Binny. I hope Alison remembers to do her teeth. She watched with interest, bent over her knees, as Harry bundled the wounded Geoff into the passenger seat. Simpson's bandage, she noticed, had come undone and hung in a frayed noose about his neck. Edward was bending down and staring at her with his mouth open. The car began to move. She could see Edward's stomach as he ran beside the window—he was holding the handle of the door, preventing it from closing. There's no room, she thought. He's too fat.

Then he was inside the car, impossibly jammed between the seats. Widnes swore and hit him in the face with his fist.

Eyes full of reproach, Edward leaned towards Binny and stretched out his arm.

"I'll never leave you," he cried.

The car gathered speed and swung round the

corner by the garage. The four occupants of the back seat lurched sideways. The door opened.

Liar, thought Binny, as Edward fell away from the car.

A woman at a window screamed, like the blast of a whistle.

DATE DUE			